CANCER ETIOLOGY, DIAGNOSIS AND TREATMENTS

ESTROGEN PREVENTION FOR BREAST CANCER

CANCER ETIOLOGY, DIAGNOSIS AND TREATMENTS

Additional books in this series can be found on Nova's website under the Series tab.

Additional e-books in this series can be found on Nova's website under the e-book tab.

Cancer Etiology, Diagnosis and Treatments

Estrogen Prevention for Breast Cancer

Zsuzsanna Suba
Editor

Nova Biomedical
New York

For permission to use material from this book please contact us:
Telephone 631-231-7269; Fax 631-231-8175
Web Site: http://www.novapublishers.com

Library of Congress Cataloging-in-Publication Data

ISBN: 978-1-62417-378-3

Library of Congress Control Number: 2012952787

Published by Nova Science Publishers, Inc. † New York

Contents

Preface

Myth of the carcinogenic capacity of estrogen emerged first at the end of 19th century when ovariectomy seemed to be advantageous for a woman against her breast cancer. From the middle of 20th century available serum hormone extractions and synthetic estrogens yielded the possibility of estrogen administration for contraception, for the treatment of anovulatory infertility and for the hormone replacement therapy of postmenopausal women. From the early 80s clinical and epidemiological studies have increasingly pointed to an elevated breast, endometrial and ovarian cancer risk of high circulating estrogen levels. Though the majority of epidemiological studies have long been suggested that estrogens play a pivotal role in mammary carcinogenesis; the exact mechanism of their carcinogenic capacity on breast epithelial cells has not yet been demonstrated till now.

Estrogen deficiency as cancer risk factor emerged first in 2007 in a study on Hungarian oral cancer cases based on the conspicuous gender and age related differences in tumor prevalence. Accumulation of postmenopausal elderly female cases among non-smoker, non-drinker oral cancer patients suggested a heretical idea: carcinogenic capacity of estrogen deficiency. This newly revealed correlation means a contradiction to the traditional concept of estrogen induced cancer in highly estrogen responsive organs. Nevertheless, the mechanism of gene regulation failures in the background of tumor initiation may not act through quite opposite pathways at different sites. Critical reevaluation of the contradictory results of hormone replacement therapy (HRT) in postmenopausal women yielded a complete conversion; estrogen deficiency may confer cancer initiation. Cancer protective effect of estrogen was prophesied even for breast cancer when methodologically strong studies avoid bias and preconception.

Since then, the anticancer capacity of estrogen was clearly justified for cancers at several sites (oral cavity, upper aerodigestive tract, lung, liver, colon, and rectum). Nevertheless, breast cancer remained as a last fortress to support the principle of the carcinogenic potency of estrogen.

A breakthrough has come in breast cancer research in 2010 in San Antonio when Canadian scientists reported on the re-evaluation of the earlier results of WHI Hormone Replacement Therapy Trial. After a proper selection of same patients, HRT use proved to be not only safe but strongly protective for breast cancer and for many other aspects of women's health.

This conversion picked up the fight for the justice of estrogen and provoked overwhelming publication activities concerning its beneficial anticancer impact even on female breast.

Recognition of the cancer protective effect of estrogen on female breast clarifies many controversies and misunderstandings in the field of experimental and clinical oncology. Deleterious interactions between estrogen deficiency and further hormonal and metabolic disorders might illuminate the apparently controversial associations of obesity, light exposure and alcohol intake with breast cancer risk.

Presumed carcinogenic impact of estrogen promoted the development of antiestrogenic compounds, which aimed the inhibition of endogenous estrogen binding to its receptor system so as to achieve a regression of hormone-related breast cancer. Antiestrogens frequently proved to be ineffective in tumor therapy and mediated severe side effects; such as vascular complications and cancer development at several sites. By contrast, reports on the estrogen treatment of advanced breast cancer cases are regularly returning from Washington and European centers and the results are encouraging.

Recently introduced principle of the anticancer potency of estrogen, may provide new insight into the etiology of mammary malignancies and leads to new strategies in the primary prevention and treatment of breast cancer.

Zsuzsanna Suba

Acknowledgements

Grateful thanks for the helpful and meritorious contribution of coauthors from Canada and United States; for Joseph Ragaz and Shayan Shakeraneh from School of Population and Public Health, University of British Columbia (Vancouver) and for Mark B. Leick and V. Craig Jordan from Georgetown Lombardi Comprehensive Cancer Center (Washington).

In: Estrogen Prevention for Breast Cancer
Editor: Zsuzsanna Suba

ISBN: 978-1-62417-378-3

Chapter I

Discovery of Estrogen Deficiency as Common Cancer Risk Factor for Highly and Moderately Estrogen Dependent Organs

Zsuzsanna Suba
National Institute of Oncology, Department of Surgical and Molecular Pathology
Budapest, Hungary

Abstract

Accumulation of non-smoker, non-drinker elderly postmenopausal female patients among smoking-associated oral cancer cases raised the plausible idea: estrogen deficiency maybe a cancer risk factor. On the other hand the extremely rare cases of young women with oral cancer regularly exhibited hormonal disorders, such as irregular menstrual cycles and infertility. Furthermore, in the history of middle-aged female oral cancer cases primary ovarian failure or complete hysterectomy were conspicuously frequent findings suggesting an estrogen deficient milieu. Also, there were many striking contradictions concerning the associations of female sexual steroids and cancer risk. Till now, breast and endometrial cancers were regarded as typically estrogen-induced tumors, particularly in post-menopausal cases. Conversely, unexplained beneficial anti-cancer effects of hormone-replacement therapy were reported against cancers at several sites even for tumors of highly hormone-responsive organs. Re-evaluation of the results of experimental and epidemiological studies, endeavoring to justify the carcinogenic capacity of estrogen, exhibited many shortcomings and controversies. Recent findings both on smoking associated and hormone related cancers added up to the same conversion; not estrogen but rather its deficiency might provoke cancer initiation. Thorough review of literary data justified that the exquisite regulatory capacity of estrogen and its surveillance on growth, development, differentiation, and metabolism are indispensable, whereas an estrogen-deficient milieu may induce a breakdown in gene-regulation. Recognition of the anticancer capacity of estrogen may provide new insights into the aetiology of malignancies and leads to new strategies for cancer prevention and cure.

Introduction

Mild or moderate estrogen deficiency is a relatively frequent, pathologic state of premenopausal women, whereas at menopause ovarian estrogen production definitely declines and serum estrogen levels show further decrease during the postmenopausal years. Conversely, pathologic, excessive estrogen production is extremely rare in women.

Distinction between cancers of moderately and highly estrogen dependent tissues is necessary, based on their different epidemiological features. Oral cancer is a typical example of moderately estrogen dependent tumors and its initiation seems to be associated with a profound estrogen loss [1]. The vast majority of malignancies of moderately estrogen dependent organs occur in the late postmenopausal years of women, when ovarian estrogen production is fairly decreased [2].

However, cancers of the highly estrogen dependent organs such as breast, usually exhibit both premenopausal and postmenopausal occurrences [3,4,5]. In premenopausal cases, marked cancer prevalence in organs with high estrogen dependence suggests that the higher hormone demand of affected organs may result in gene regulation disorders even in mildly or moderately estrogen deficient milieu [6].

In spite of the different epidemiological data of these two groups of cancers the mechanism of gene regulation disorder in the background of tumor initiation cannot act through quite opposite pathways. Many literary data justify that insulin resistance, obesity and type-2 diabetes are in similarly close association with cancer risk of both highly and moderately estrogen dependent organs [7]. Conversely, the newly revealed association between estrogen deficiency and oral cancer risk indicates a contradiction to the traditional concept of estrogen induced breast cancer. This contradiction may raise the plausible question whether increased or decreased serum estrogen levels might be the common risk factors for cancers of highly and moderately estrogen dependent organs?

Risk Factors for Cancers of Highly Hormone Related Organs

Cancers of highly estrogen dependent organs are in the forefront of tumors as they are regarded as hormone associated ones. They have multicausal origin, however, in the past decades female sexual steroids, especially estrogens were presumed to be important etiologic factors. The incidence rate of so-called hormone dependent tumors such as breast, endometrial and ovarian cancers is highest in the industrialized countries and much lower in the developing countries, with a highest to lowest ratio of 20:1 [8].

Breast tumors are important subjects of cancer research as they are the most frequent cancers in the women of the Western world. Marked geographic differences in breast cancer morbidity and mortality seem to be environmental rather than genetic in origin [3]. As higher economic development is in close correlation with higher prevalence of insulin resistance and obesity, differences in breast cancer incidence may be partially associated with the epidemiological features of metabolic diseases.

Traditional concept of the carcinogenic capacity of the female sex steroid hormones was based on the epidemiological data of breast cancer cases [9,10,11,12]. *Endogenous estrogen*was regarded as a risk for breast cancer even in case of slightly elevated circulatory level [9,13,14,15]. *Exogenous estrogens* administered alone or in combination with progestin were found also to be risk factors for breast cancer [16,17,18,19]. Results of the hormone replacement therapy (HRT) of postmenopausal women supported the relative breast cancer risk in summarized population based epidemiological studies [20]. Further literary data suggested that HRT use for more than 5-10 years means an increased relative risk for mammary malignancies [21].

Breast cancer is a tumor of fairly hormone dependent tissue, exhibiting both premenopausal and postmenopausal manifestations even without exogenous estrogen treatment [4]. Epidemiological observations can hardly be explained by the carcinogenic capacity of the elevated level of female sexual steroids, especially in postmenopausal cases. Moreover, as the majority of malignancies, breast cancer is also a multicausal tumor with strong genetic associations.

Risk factors established or suspected to be associated with breast cancer are numerous [22]. Family history and genetic disposition, lifestyle including diet, physical exercise, smoking, excessive alcohol consumption and individual hormonal and reproductive factors all markedly influence the incidence of this tumor. Recently, insulin resistant states such as obesity, elevated fasting glucose, metabolic syndrome and type-2 diabetes are also regarded as strong risk factors for breast cancer [23]. Thus hormone replacement therapy (HRT) is only one of a broad range of factors for which an inconsistent association with breast cancer of postmenopausal cases has been found.

Endometrial cancer is the most common invasive malignancy of the female genital tract with both pre- and postmenopausal variants as well [24]. Known risk factors associated with increased risk for endometrial cancer are also numerous. Among others old age, metabolic syndrome, type-2 diabetes, obesity, nulliparity, alcohol use, oral contraception and HRT use are regarded as risks for endometrial malignancies [25,26].

Hyperestrogenism is regarded as a causal factor for endometrial hyperplasia, which may be the predecessor of endometrial adenocarcinoma [27]. Many epidemiologists have accepted exogenous estrogen administration as a risk factor for human endometrial cancer [28,29,30]. Increased cancer risk was established with increasing estrogen doses and with the longer duration of treatment [31].

Literary data on the endometrial cancer risk by oral contraception show controversial results. Some authors suggested a decreased cancer risk of highly hormone dependent organs associated with oral contraception explained by a decreased cumulative number of ovulations [31,32]. Recently, insulin resistance has been in the forefront as risk for endometrial carcinoma. Drugs, used for the treatment of type-2 diabetes, are important candidates for prevention and possible treatment of endometrial carcinoma [33].

A dualistic model of endometrial carcinogenesis was proposed earlier [34], whith possible importance in the evaluation of associations of HRT with endometrial cancer. According to this concept, there are two main types of endometrial carcinomas in correlation with circulatory estrogen supply. The first type is a slowly spreading, highly differentiated form, supposedly developing in association with excessive estrogen stimulation (type I). The second type is a more aggressive variant considered to arise in a relatively estrogen-deficient milieu of elderly women (type II)! The type I form of endometrial cancer, which may be potentially associated with HRT use, is less aggressive, with a 5-year survival rate of 70-80% [35]. The type II, poorly differentiated endometrial carcinoma affects older women and the 5-year survival rate is shorter or about 60%.

Recently, a third type of mucinous endometrial carcinoma has been associated with the use of tamoxifen, which is an estrogen antagonist drug used against estrogen receptor positive breast cancers [26,36]. An important parallelism between breast and endometrial cancers is that only the estrogen receptor positive, highly differentiated, slow growing forms have been assumed to have associations with HRT use [26,37].

Ovarian cancer represents about 30% of all malignancies of the female genital tract. The age adjusted incidence rates vary from <2/100 000 women in most of Southeast Asia and Africa to >15/100 000 cases in Northern and Eastern Europe [8]. The economically advanced countries of North America and Europe show the highest rates.

In the USA an increased risk of ovarian cancer mortality was associated with postmenopausal estrogen use based on a large prospective study [38]. A collaborative reanalysis of European studies found a relative risk of ovarian cancer related to ever use of HRT [39]. Recently, in a cohort study a strong relationship was established between duration of estrogen therapy and risk of ovarian cancer [40].

The incidence of ovarian cancer shows a steady increase with age. Reduced risk of the disease is consistently associated with high parity and oral contraceptive use [35]. Energy rich diet and insulin resistance have also been related to ovarian cancer [41].

In conclusion, the carcinogenic capacity of circulating estrogens became a prevailing concept at the turn of the millennium, particularly in association with the malignancies of highly hormone dependent organs [42].

Controversial Associations of Hormone Replacement Therapy and Cancer Risk

Hormone replacement therapy (HRT) in postmenopausal women has been fairly widespread in the economically developed countries in the past decades. These cases supply excellent possibilities to study the associations between female sexual steroid hormones and tumor incidence. Till now, the prevailing concept is that HRT is associated with an increased prevalence of gynecological cancers [12,43,44].

However, recent clinical studies on HRT use in postmenopausal women yielded unexpected and fairly controversial associations with malignancies [45,46]. Unexplained, beneficial anticancer effects of HRT use were reported against *gastric,oral, esophageal,colorectal, cervical, liver and lung cancers* [12,44,47,48,49,50,51,52] and there are also contradictory results concerning the associations of HRT and highly hormone dependent cancers[37,53,54].

Urinary bladder cancer is a typically smoking associated tumor and its risk is three to four times higher in men than in women [55]. Striking contradictions have been published concerning the associations between HRT and urinary bladder cancer. Among HRT user women an excess risk was found for bladder cancer in a case-control study [44]. Other authors could not justify any association of hormone related factors with bladder cancer incidence in women [56]. However, in a follow up study, estrogen deficiency such as postmenopausal status and a short reproductive period caused by menopause at young age did unfavorably affect the risk for bladder cancer in women [57].

Just as urinary bladder cancer, *upper aerodigestive tract tumors* are strongly smoking associated too, and their incidence also shows a high male to female ratio. Cancer incidence at these sites exhibits controversial associations with HRT use as well. Laryngeal cancer is the neoplasm with the largest male to female sex ratio in most populations. In a case-control study on women with laryngeal cancer, menstrual and hormonal factors did not appear to have a consistent role in laryngeal carcinogenesis [58].

Conversely, prospective clinical studies justified a protective role of long term HRT (48 months) against smoking associated tumors, such as oral, laryngeal and pharyngeal cancers among current smokers, but did not affect the tumor incidence among non-smokers[48]. The authors supposed that HRT postpones rather than prevents the smoking associated cancers by a transitory maintenance of epithelial thickness and integrity in the upper aero-digestive tract, which may counteract exogenous carcinogenic agents. In a Hungarian case control study late menopause showed a negative, whereas postmenopausal state a positive association with oral cancer risk in women [1]. Considering the results of Hungarian studies on oral cancer cases systemic hormonal effects of HRT use may both prevent and postpone the induction of oral cancer. Associations of hormonal factors and upper digestive tract cancer risk exhibited beneficial anticancer effect of older age at menopause and postmenopausal estrogen therapy [59]. These findings support the beneficial effect of good hormonal equilibrium against cancer risk.

Lung cancer is also highly smoking-associated tumor and its incidence exhibits high male to female ratio. Studies on correlations between HRT and lung cancer risk in women have reported controversial associations. HRT was associated with decreased survival in women with lung cancer [60]. Nevertheless, HRT use in postmenopausal women was associated with reduced lung cancer risk, particularly after longer duration [61]. Recently, HRT was found to be associated with reduced risk for lung cancer independent of smoking status; however, this association was strongest among never smokers [50].

HRT also has anticancer capacities at other tumor sites other than the upper aero-digestive tract such as in *stomach, colon, liver and cervix* [44,49,51,52], which can hardly be explained by a local defense mechanism against tobacco products and exogenous carcinogenic agents. HRT probably exerts this advantageous effect by means of its systemic metabolic and hormonal pathways. Late menopause and longer duration of fertile life seems to correlate with a reduced risk for gastric cancer [52].

Epidemiological evidences suggest that HRT is associated with a small but substantial increase in breast cancer risk among postmenopausal women [43]. Nevertheless, some of the clinical studies failed to identify any association between increased serum hormone levels and breast cancer [62,63]. Though HRT was regarded as breast cancer risk factor from 10 studies reviewed, only 5 showed statistically significant positive association between hormone treatment and breast cancer risk whereas, the other 5 studies could not justify this correlation [20]. In a recent study, long lasting treatment with conjugated equine estrogens did not increase breast cancer incidence in postmenopausal women with prior hysterectomy [64]. Moreover, in the Women's Health Initiative randomised trials on postmenopausal women with prior hysterectomy estrogen treatment was associated with a marked reduction in breast cancer risk [54,65,66]. Authors could not explain these unexpected findings though hysterectomy means a uniformly increased risk for women included into this study.

Positive correlation between HRT and endometrial cancer has been firmly established by epidemiological studies [28,29,30,43]. An increased risk was established with increasing doses of estrogen as well as with the length of treatment [17]. Conversely, an increased risk for endometrial cancer has not been justified in association with HRT either by the Women's Health Initiative (WHI) randomised trial [53] or by the Heart and Estrogen/Progestin Replacement Study (HERS) [67]. Moreover, further studies could justify even a decreased risk for endometrial cancer in postmenopausal women with HRT use [33].

Associations between HRT and *ovarian cancer* are fairly controversial [43]. A review of 20 studies on ovarian cancer reached no satisfactory conclusion concerning HRT risk for this tumor [68]. Five of these studies described a slightly elevated ovarian cancer risk in HRT users, whereas the other 15 studies did not. Recently, further doubts concerning associations between HRT use and ovarian cancer risk have emerged [69].

All these controversial correlations between HRT use and cancer risk for both smoking associated and hormone related tumors suggest that a thorough revision of the concept concerning the carcinogenic capacity of estrogen would be necessary.

Shortcomings of Studies on the Correlations between HRT Use and Cancer Risk

The postmenopausal period in women is a physiological model for studies on the hormonal, metabolic and gene regulation changes associated with estrogen deficiency. In healthy postmenopausal women there are physiological mechanisms to adapt to the gradual loss of estrogen signals. However, this new equilibrium comprises many risks and traps for slipping out of the regular metabolic and hormonal pathways.

An abrupt decrease in estrogen hormone levels either after a natural or an artificial menopause may cause gene regulation disturbances not only in the female reproductive system but also in many other organs. Radical or subtotal hysterectomy in premenopausal women results in a sudden, definite loss of ovarian estrogen synthesis and may cause severe consequences, especially without HRT use. Spontaneous or induced abortion also causes a transitory but shocking fall in the hormone levels.

In clinical practice about 40% of women have severe menopausal complaints usually requiring medical help [70]. Menopausal complaints are not only unpleasant, bothering symptoms but suggest thorough disorders of adaptation to estrogen loss and a possibility for altered gene regulation. The hormonal alterations affect the general health of the women, as they are risks for both cardiovascular diseases and malignancies. If estrogen deficiency is regarded as a risk for cancers these patients have a greater cancer risk in their later life as compared with women who have gradually, asymptomatically lost their estrogen signals and have no need for HRT use. These considerations suggest that cancer risk in aged women, among other factors, may depend on their endogenous hormonal characteristics, their menopausal process and on HRT use in their history.

Correct evaluation of correlations between HRT use and cancer risk requires strict selection of the patients included, proper length of the observational period and awareness of the estrogen receptor positivity of tumors.

Selection of the Patients for HRT Studies

Cancers are multicausal diseases, and the carcinogenic capacity of the physiological levels of female sexual steroids is hardly, if at all justifiable. The investigation of HRT use, as a supposed cancer risk factor on pooled, unselected population of women is misleading.

Supposedly, neither the hormone treated nor the untreated groups of women involved in HRT studies are homogenous. The marked differences in menopausal processes in women and their various effects on gene regulation may partially explain the controversies concerning the associations of HRT and cancer.

Correlations between HRT use and breast cancer risk are usually examined in two groups of involved women; with and without hormone treatment, disregarding their individual hormonal and reproductive differences and other known or suspected risk factors. In these studies the majority of HRT user women may be assumed to have severe postmenopausal complaints in connection with a failure of the adaptation mechanisms. However, women without hormone treatment may have predominantly uneventful perimenopausal period due to their good adaptation. Consequently, the epidemiological studies on breast cancer risk of HRT users reflect an additive effect of the endogenous hormonal features of the HRT user population and of their hormone treatment.

A collaborative re-analysis was performed on data from 51 epidemiological studies dealing mainly with single estrogen substitution [71]. The overall relative risk for breast cancer was as low as 1.14 when HRT users were compared with never users. The increase in the risk was very small but significant because of the great number of examined cases. However, a WHI publication could find no risk for breast cancer among women who used estrogen alone, even unopposed estrogen treatment was associated with a marked reduction in breast cancer risk (HR: 0.77) [54]. The WHI authors suggested that this reduction in breast cancer risk associated to HRT requires further investigation. This valuable study seems to be a stretching force against the old frame of carcinogenicity of estrogen.

Small differences in breast cancer risk between HRT user and untreated populations of women - even advantageously decreased breast cancer risk as a result of one-armed estrogen treatment - raise the possibility of bias and improper patient selection in the majority of studies [6].

How can we explain the results of the widespread epidemiological studies, which support the slightly but consequently higher breast cancer risk in postmenopausal women with HRT use as compared with untreated cases?

Estrogen deficiency seems to be a cancer risk factor, especially for highly estrogen dependent organs. Women belonging to the group of HRT users supposedly have severe postmenopausal complaints based on failure of their adaptation. Consequently, HRT users have a higher risk for breast cancer initiation as compared with complaint-free women without treatment.

Presumably, the beneficial effect of HRT use may decrease the rate of new cancer initiation in postmenopausal women. However, the pre-existing subclinical cancers induced by the pre- or perimenopausal hormonal disorders cannot be completely destroyed. Consequently, an elevated breast cancer incidence may remain in the group of endangered women with severe endogenous hormone deficiency and/or defective adaptation mechanism in spite of HRT use. These considerations may explain the slightly but consequently elevated breast cancer risk among HRT users as compared with untreated women with physiological adaptation.

Furthermore, the estrogen deficiency theory justifies that in a methodologically stronger WHI study an unexpected, beneficial effect of HRT use against breast cancer was observed [54]. One-armed HRT was applied on 10 793 women with prior hysterectomy by conjugated estrogen and it was found to be associated with reduction of breast cancer risk. This result justifies the importance of selection of homogenously endangered patients for epidemiological studies and supports the protective role of estrogen against breast cancer.

The effects of adaptation disorders on breast cancer risk should be prospectively studied via comparison of untreated patients with and without postmenopausal complaints. Moreover, associations of HRT use and breast cancer risk might be correctly examined if the cases and controls have similar menopausal and reproductive histories and their further risk factors are also matched.

Dynamics of Cancer Growths and the Length of Observational Period

Dynamics of breast cancer initiation and promotion is still poorly understood [72,73,74,75]. Thus, firm causal conclusions cannot be established from the associations between hormone treatment and breast cancer found on inhomogeneous female populations.

Studies on HRT user women failed to clarify whether hormone treatment apparently stimulates induction of cancers de novo by initiating mutations, or facilitates the growth of pre-existing, small tumors [37].

The tumor doubling time (TDT) concept is useful for assessment of the duration of prediagnostic stage of cancers. It is defined as the time for a tumor volume or cell number to double once [76]. TDT depends on many variables such as rate of cell division, proportion of actively dividing cells, rate of apoptoses, angiogenetic potential, intermitotic interval, shedding of tumor cells, ratio of tumor and stromal cells and so on. These numerous factors explain the wide range of estimations of TDT in breast cancer [77,78]. Current data show that a median TDT for human cancers may be 50-100 days [76].

A size of 1 cm in diameter is more or less the smallest tumor to be diagnosed clinically. This corresponds to rough and ready 10^9 cells but this number depends strongly on the tumor cell size [78]. This means that on average at least 1750-3500 days (5-10 years) are necessary from the initial mutation to a clinically and/or mammographically detectable tumor mass [79]. However, this calculation is true for a tumor only in case of ideal circumstances and does not consider the cell loss by apoptosis, death and shedding [76].Further, there are no data concerning the time demand of the transition from an intraepithelial, non-invasive cancer to an invasive one, which will further prolong the period from tumor initiation to clinical cancer diagnosis [37]. In reality, the estimated time from initiation to a diagnosable cancer might be much longer than 5-10 years.

Considering the theories on tumor growth dynamics, the presumable time between supposed initiation of breast tumors by HRT and clinical detection seems to be at least 10 years or even longer [78]. All the studies showing associations between HRT and breast cancer are based on far shorter observational periods.

Awareness of Estrogen Receptor Positivity of Cancers

Mechanisms of initiation versus promotion of hormone dependent cancers, particularly breast cancer, are only scarcely understood. A widespread theory is that hormonal influence of breast cancer is necessary from the primordial mutation to clinical cancer diagnosis after many years [67].

The pathophysiological prerequisite for the initiation and progression of hormoneinduced cancer in postmenopausal women and its association with HRT use is the presence of active estrogen receptors in the target tissues [37]. However, it is a well-known fact that estrogen receptor expression is fairly different in breast cancers and there are also receptor-negative tumors. Unfortunately, the studies, which formed the current view on the HRT-induced cancer risk, did not incorporate biochemical or immunohistochemical data to clarify levels of estrogen receptor expression of breast cancers. These shortcomings may also explain the controversial associations of HRT and breast cancer risk and the results become questionable.

Doubts concerning HRT induced cancer initiation. Majority of breast cancers detected in association with HRT use are histologically well differentiated and have a relatively good prognosis [37]. These are usually slowly growing cancers and do not metastasize early. Generally, the low-grade breast cancers with low malignancy are estrogen receptor positive. As hormone receptors are presumably the prerequisites for the theoretical impact of HRT use on breast cancer initiation, only the differentiated, receptor positive cancers with slow progression may be associated with hormonal influences.

However, initiation of both ER-positive and ER-negative breast cancers may be equally possible based on the estrogen deficiency theory. Gene regulation disturbance caused by estrogen loss does not require normal ER signals; in contrast, overwhelming growth factor activities become predominant versus non-liganded, altered ERs. In this manner estrogen deficiency may induce highly differentiated, receptor-positive or poorly differentiated receptor-negative cancers.

ER-positive breast cancers are predominantly slow growing tumors requiring longer period between presumed HRT-induced initiation and clinical cancer diagnosis as compared with undifferentiated, receptor negative ones. Consequently, for hormone receptor positive, highly differentiated cancers an even much longer observational period would be necessary to establish the correlation between HRT use and breast cancer risk.

By contrast, estrogen deficiency induced breast cancer may be initiated in the pre- or perimenopausal period by moderate estrogen loss previous to the beginning of HRT. At menopause a further, abrupt decrease of estrogen level may provoke postmenopausal complaints and at the same time, faster growth of the pre-existing cancer. However, HRT use will alleviate the complaints and diminish the aggressivity of early cancer. This explanation illuminates both the possibility of clinical cancer diagnosis as early as after 4-5 years of HRT use and the lower aggressivity of cancers associated with hormone treatment.

Doubts concerning HRT induced cancer promotion. Dietel et al. proposed that as the observation time of women with HRT use is not long enough, hormones may not initiate but may perhaps accelerate the tumor growth leading to an earlier clinical discovery [37]. A contradictory result with HRT associated promotion of breast cancer is the slower growth, reduced aggressivity of tumors and longer survival among HRT user women as compared with those who did not take HRT. Nevertheless, as only hormone dependent tumors may be affected by HRT and hormone receptor expression means a higher differentiation of breast cancers, it is not probable that hormone treatment induces dedifferentiation and more rapid progression of tumors.

Cancer initiation and promotion are generally not contradictory processes. There are many factors, including hormonal signals, which may induce both cancer initiation and promotion. Increased rates of tumor initiation and progression have been observed in compensatory hyperinsulinemia associated with insulin resistance. Elevated insulin and concomitantly elevated IGF levels are proven risk factors for both breast cancer initiation and progression [23]. In case of another hormone, such as estrogen, an inverse effect on tumor initiation as compared with tumor promotion is hardly justifiable.

Estrogen Deficiency and Cancer Risk in Postmenopausal Women

Cancer development requires many years from initiation to clinical appearance, and this is valid also for estrogen deficient postmenopausal women, especially if the main exogenous cancer risk factors are missing. The majority of postmenopausal cancers may be initiated at the perimenopausal or postmenopausal estrogen deficient period and the clinical manifestation occurs much later. As the average age at menopause is about 50 years in Hungary, the age above 60 may be especially dangerous for clinical appearance of malignancies at moderately estrogen dependent sites in women [1].

Smoking associated tumors can be regarded as typically *moderately estrogen dependent malignancies* such as cancers of the oral cavity, pharynx, larynx, lung and urinary bladder. Their incidence exhibits very high male to female ratios and has controversial correlations with HRT use. Recent literary data support that postmenopausal hormone therapy seems to have advantageous anticancer impact on these types of cancers [6]. These observations suggest that estrogen loss in postmenopausal women may have crucial role in development of smoking-related cancers, which seems to be independent of smoking habits [1,81,82].

Oral cancer is a typically smoking-associated tumor with high male to female ratio and is regarded as a moderately hormone dependent cancer type. The almost exclusively *postmenopausal state* of female oral cancer patients suggests that estrogen deficiency has crucial role in the development of this tumor [1,81]. The length of the interval between menopause and tumor onset proved also to be decisive factor in the clinical appearance of oral cancer. A fairly long mean interval between menopause of oral cancer cases and tumor diagnosis (near 17 years) suggested an important role of estrogen deprivation in oral cancer initiation. The longer theperiod of estrogen deficiency the higher the possibility of postmenopausal tumor manifestation.

An early menopause, such as premature ovarian failure under 40 years of age or premenopausal hysterectomy with or without ovariectomy means a *shorter hormonally activereproductive period* and may have thorough consequences affecting gene regulation. A significantly higher ratio of young age (<45 yrs) at menopause among the female oral cancer cases as compared with the age-matched tumor-free controls was demonstrated [1].

Moreover, a *sudden loss of the estrogen signal* may be an especially dangerous shock for the regulatory mechanisms both in the highly and moderately estrogen dependent organs.

Hysterectomy with or without ovariectomy proved to be a high risk factor for oral cancer among women in our epidemiological study [1,81].

Cancers of the highly estrogen dependent organs such as breast cancer may also occur in older postmenopausal cases. In these women a good hormonal equilibrium may be presumed during their reproductive period, which defends the highly hormone dependent organs from cancer initiation. The first shock of estrogen loss arises in the perimenopausal period, which may serve as cancer initiator. However, the continuously decreasing ovarian estrogen synthesis during postmenopausal life may be a sword of Damocles for all organs.

Moderate Estrogen Deficiency and Cancer Risk in Premenopausal Women

Carcinogenic effects of marked estrogen deficiency may easily be studied in women, since their life is clearly separated into premenopausal and postmenopausal periods. However, the long-term systemic effects of mildly or moderately decreased estrogen levels in premenopausal women maybe hard to clarify.

In premenopausal women there are many pathological states predisposing to mild or moderate estrogen deficiency. Ovarian insufficiency may result in long or irregular menstrual cycles and unexplained infertility. Chronic anovulation and ovulatory dysfunction were found also to be associated with increased prevalence of endometrial cancer [83]. Spontaneous and induced abortions provoke sudden decrease of the highly elevated estrogen level and may be regarded as transitory periods with increased inclination to disorders of gene regulation. Literary data are controversial concerning the associations of abortion and breast cancer risk; however, late termination of pregnancy at abortion seems to be a high risk for breast cancer [84]. Immunosuppressive therapy against autoimmune diseases, cancer or rejection reaction in organ transplantation cases may also induce ovarian insufficiency and risk for development of malignancies.

Polycystic ovarian syndrome (PCOS) is a complex disorder that is presumably caused by a large number of different genetic abnormalities. PCOS is the most common endocrinopathy of women in the reproductive age [85,86,87]. PCOS seems to be a pathological model of hormonal and metabolic alterations of postmenopausal status in premenopausal women. It may usually be manifested by menstrual disorders, anovulation, infertility, hirsutism and obesity and means a conspicuously increased risk for cancers at highly estrogen dependent sites [85,86,88].

Some authors suppose that unopposed estrogen levels continuously stimulate ERs in women with PCOS, which maybe a risk for endometrial and breast cancers [86]. However, insulin resistance and hyperinsulinemia in patients with PCOS are associated with high ovarian androgen synthesis and estrogen deficiency [89].

Infertility is the most sensitive indicator of hormonal disorders in symptom-free women. PCOS cases diagnosed among adolescents suggest that the disease may develop insidiously during puberty rather than at a later time of presentation of infertility [87]. Consequently, hormonal insufficiency may be long lasting enough to promote cancer development in the young adulthood of affected women.

PCOS has a great significance as latent, undiagnosed cases are relatively numerous among the female population [90,91]. If the diagnosis is based on the morphological findings of ovarian pathology at either surgery or ultrasonography, then up to 20% of unselected women have been reported to be affected [90,92]. Or about 25% of these women have no clinical symptoms although many do have laboratory findings suggesting endocrinological and metabolic disturbances associated with PCOS such as hyperandrogenism and hyperinsulinemia [23].

PCOS-associated endocrine alterations mean risk factors for breast and gynecological cancers. In otherwise healthy, young premenopausal patients with unexpected malignancies a thorough endocrinological examination should be performed.

Conspicuous Differences between Cancer Epidemiology of Highly and Moderately Estrogen Dependent Organs

Epidemiological studies on the incidence rate of moderately estrogen dependent cancers provide the possibility to compare the data of the two genders, whereas in case of highly hormone dependent cancers of women this advantage is excluded.

The most important source of misunderstandings and misinterpretations in the epidemiology of highly estrogen dependent breast cancer may be that its exhibition is almost exclusively restricted to one gender. On the contrary, in case of the moderately hormone dependent oral cancer, gender-related epidemiological differences and their trends have raised many questions to be answered [93]. Moreover, the gender-related differences in oral cancer epidemiology served as leaders on the route from smoking associated cancers to the discovery of estrogen deficiency induced carcinogenesis.

Recently estrogen and its receptors are regarded as pivotal gene regulators affecting cell growth, proliferation, differentiation and metabolism [94]. Cells of all tissues and organs have estrogen receptors with variable expression levels and they are deeply influenced by estrogen receptor signal induced mechanisms even out of the female genital tract. Therefore, assumption of a strict distinction or even inverse mechanisms between carcinogenesis in highly and moderately estrogen dependent organs is not reasonable.

Cancers of the *highly estrogen dependent breast, endometrium and ovary* have certain special characteristics even without exogenous hormone treatment. They have no sharp distinction concerning the incidence rate between premenopausal and postmenopausal cases.

Epidemiological data on cancers of the highly estrogen dependent organs show a relatively wide range of ages among patients. Moreover, among breast cancer cases at least 25-30% of the affected women are premenopausal [3]. Recently, in a prospective study on breast cancer cases over than 50% of the patients were premenopausal [4]. These data suggest that for the highly estrogen dependent organs even a mild or moderate estrogen deficiency in young, premenopausal cases is enough to initiate gene regulation disorders. Breast cancer, which is a typical example of cancers of the highly hormone related tissues, is quite uncommon in women younger than 30 years of age. Thereafter, the breast cancer risk steadily increases throughout life and after menopause the upward slope of the curve is much less steep [3]. Endometrial cancer may also occur in young women and up to 30% of the cases may be premenopausal [5].

These epidemiological data seem to support the carcinogenic capacity of moderate estrogen deficiency in young, premenopausal cases affecting both tumor initiation and promotion. Development of decreased or instable estrogen levels may be originated in adolescence and it may be completely symptom-free apart from fertility problems. Organs with high estrogen demand may be disturbed in their gene regulation at very young ages by hormonal disorders. Insidious, mild estrogen deficiency in puberty may result in development of diagnosable breast, endometrial or ovarian tumor in young adults.

Later, the disorders of the hormonal equilibrium show a continuously increasing prevalence with age. Transitory or definite estrogen loss in the reproductive period caused by endogenous ovarian insufficiency, abortions, therapeutic measures or other causes may result in increasing prevalence of cancers in the highly hormone dependent organs.

Among premenopausal PCOS cases with hormonal disorders an increased prevalence of cancers could be observed preferentially in the breast, endometrium and ovary [85,86,88,95]. In a mortality study on patients with PCOS breast cancer proved to be the leading cause of death [85].

During the postmenopausal years further increase of breast cancer incidence can be observed. Initiation of breast tumors diagnosed in cases within 1-5 years after menopause may not be associated with either the exact date of the last menstruation or with HRT use. Tumor induction in these cases may be originated from a long lasting pre- or perimenopausal hormonal deficiency. Moreover, the postmenopausal abrupt decrease of estrogen levels may help the faster growth of a pre-existing, subclinical cancer.

Cancers of the *moderately estrogen dependent organs* occur typically in older women [2] who are supposedly postmenopausal suggestive of a profound estrogen loss in association with initiation of these tumors. Moderately estrogen dependent cancers show striking differences in prevalence and age related distribution in the two genders. The male to female ratios of oral cancer showed a conspicuous dromedary-shape curve when studied in different age groups (Figure 1).

Shockingly young oral cancer cases less than 30 years of age are extremely rare. Among them the effect of traditional, exogenous risk factors such as excessive alcohol intake or tobacco may be excluded, and a low male to female ratio or even predominance of female cases could be observed [93].

In young women oral cancer initiation requires more profound estrogen deficiency from their adolescence as compared with the highly estrogen dependent cancers. As oral cancer has a multicausal origin, a further possibility is the coexistence of mild estrogen deficiency with other non-traditional cancer risk factors.

Similar, estrogen deficient states are probably extremely rare in young boys; theoretically it is rather androgen excess, which may provoke their gene regulation disorders. These differences in hormonal disorders may explain the equalization of the male to female ratio of oral cancer among cases less than 30 years of age.

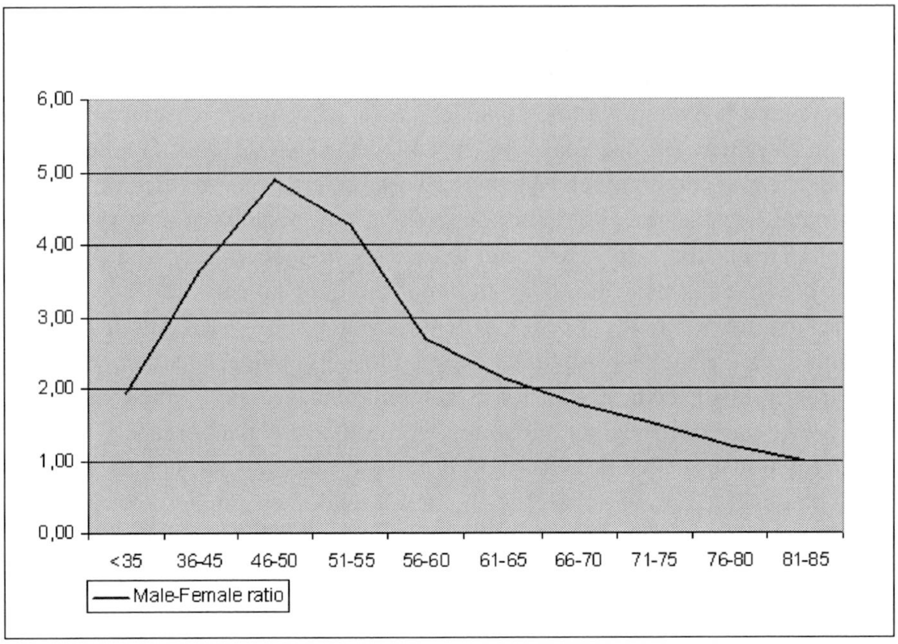

Figure 1. Male to female ratio of oral cancer patients depending on their age shows a dromedary like curve and a steep decline begins at 51-55 years of age.

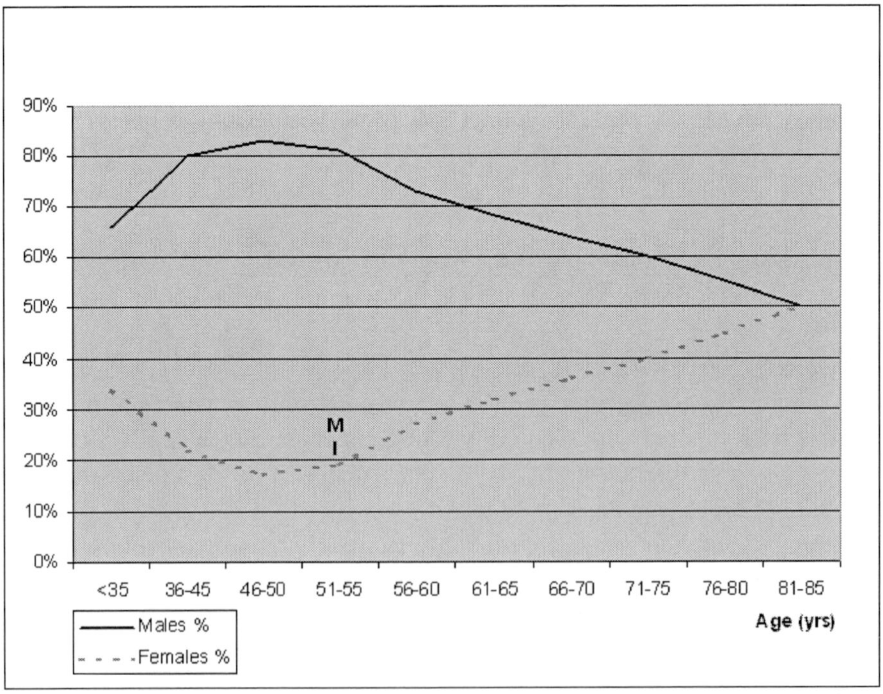

Figure 2.Percentage of male and female cases among oral cancer patients depending on their age. Between 40 and 60 years of age the male to female ratio is constantly high. At mean age of menopause (M) an increasing trend of cancer incidence among females but a decreasing trend among males can be observed.

Oral cancer incidence in adult and middle aged female cases (between 40-60 yrs) is rare as healthy women in their reproductive period enjoy the protective effect of female sexual steroids against cancers. Moreover, moderately estrogen dependent cancers are rarely associated with mild hormonal disorders. Consequently, oral cancer cases between the ages of 40 and 60 exhibit the highest male to female ratio because of the low incidence rate of women. As clinical cancer diagnosis from perimenopausal tumor initiation requires at least 10 years or more, the male to female ratio of diagnosable oral cancer remains high till the age of early 60s.

However, above the age of 60, or about 10 years after the mean age at menopause a sharply increasing ratio of female oral cancer cases as compared with males justifies the tumor inductive effect of a sudden estrogen decrease at menopause. Percentage of male and female cases among oral cancer patients depending on their age exhibits characteristic fish-shaped curves (Figure 2). These age-dependent, gender related differences in oral cancer prevalence might plausibly derive from the coarse hormonal changes between the reproductive and postmenopausal periods of women [6].

Extraovarian Estrogen Synthesis

There are recently clarified possibilities for extraovarian estrogen synthesis in postmenopausal women. In premenopausal women and estrous animals, the principal source of estradiol is ovarian, however, during reproductive senescence a significant amount of estradiol is produced extragonadally.

Female sexual steroids may be synthesized from precursor steroids by aromatase enzyme activity in many cell and tissue types included vascular endothelium, bone, brain, breast and endometrium [30,96,97,98]. Surprisingly, these are the very tissues evidently endangered by an estrogen deficient milieu and the severe consequences are cardiovascular disease, osteoporosis and ischemic injuries of the central nervous system. Similarly, aromatase activity and extragonadal estrogen synthesis in the highly estrogen dependent breast and endometrium suggest important defensive roles in postmenopausal women against cancer initiation.

Some authors regarded estrogen accumulation in the breast tissue of postmenopausal women as justification of hormone induced carcinogenesis in estrogen deficient cases [21]. However, it is not probable that a biological process serves as a facilitation of cancer development. Rather, it may be a defensive mechanism, as highly estrogen dependent tissues have increased inclination to cancer initiation in a hormone deficient milieu.

Estrogen Deficiency in Men

In men, the metabolic importance of estrogen milieu has been newly recognized. Recently, the role of sexual steroid equilibrium seems to be also essential in male physiology [99].

Complete estrogen deficiency in men is extremely rare such as aromatase deficiency and estrogen resistance [100,101]. Examinations on these sporadic male cases resulted in striking findings concerning metabolic disorders, such as severe type-2 diabetes being resistant to usual therapy. In these totally estrogen deficient male cases type-2 diabetes may be treated by estrogen administration. Of course, these sporadic estrogen deficient male cases cannot supply any information concerning the long-term effects, even the carcinogenicity of their hormonal disorder.

Currently, the pathophysiological effects of moderate estrogen deficiency in men and its consequences are quite obscure. Based on the more conspicuous findings found in female cases, a disturbed equilibrium of sexual steroids and especially estrogen deficiency may also be important cancer risk factor in men.

Conclusion

The novel hypothesis of estrogen deficiency as a cancer risk factor may explain the controversial associations between estrogen and cancer risk. It gives an explanation as to how typically smoking associated tumors could be initiated without a smoking history and how cancers related to estrogen deficiency could be induced both in moderately and highly estrogen dependent organs. The new findings both on smoking associated and hormone related cancers might lead to the same conversion; not estrogen but rather its deficiency may provoke cancer initiation. Recognition of the anticancer capacity of estrogen may provide new insights into the aetiology of malignancies and leads to new strategies for cancer prevention and cure.

References

[1] SubaZs. Gender-related hormonal risk factors for oral cancer. *Pathol.Oncol. Res.* 13:195-202, 2007.

[2] Kumar V, Abbas AK, Fausto N, Mitchell RN: *Robbins Basic Pathology*. 8th edition Saunders Elsevier 2007.

[3] Montag A, Kumar V. The female genital system and breast Chapter 19 In: Kumar V, Abbas AK, Fausto N, Mitchell RN: Rob*bins Basic Pathology*. 8th edition Saunders Elsevier 2007.

[4] Muti P, Quattrin T, Grant BJB et al. Fasting glucose is a risk factor for breast cancer. *Cancer Epidemiol.Biomark. and Prev.* 11:1361-1368, 2002.

[5] Soliman PT, Oh JC, Schmeler KM, Sun CC, Slomovitz BM, Gershenson DM, Burke TW, Lu KH. Risk factors for young premenopausal women with endometrial cancer. *Obstet. Gynecol.* 105:575-580, 2005.

[6] SubaZs. Re-evaluation of the epidemiological associations of female sexual steroids and cancer risk. Chapter 6. In: *Estrogen versus cancer*. Nova Science Publishers, Inc. New York, 2009.

[7] SubaZs. Insulin resistance, hyperinsulinemia and cancer risk. Chapter 2. In: *Estrogen versus cancer*. Nova Science Publishers, Inc. New York, 2009.

[8] American Institute for Cancer Research /World cancer Research Fund Food, nutrition and the prevention of cancer: a global perspective. American Institute of Cancer Research, Washington, DC 252-287, 2002.

[9] Key TJ, Applyby PN, Reeves GK. Body mass index, serum sex hormones and breast cancer risk in postmenopausal women. *J. Natl.Cancer Inst.* 95:1218-1226, 2003.

[10] Berrino F, Muti P, Micheli A, Bolelli G, Krogh V, Sciajno R et al. Serum sex hormon levels after menopause and subsequent breast cancer. *J. Natl. Cancer Inst.* 88:291-296, 1996.

[11] Kabuto M, Akiba S, Stevens RG, Neriishi K, Land CE. A prospective study of estradiol and breast cancer in Japanese women. *Cancer Epidemiol.Biomark.and Prev.*9:575-579, 2000.

[12] La Vecchia C, Brinton LA, McTiernan A. Menopause, hormone replacement therapy and cancer. *Maturitas.* 39:97-115, 2001.

[13] Feigelson HS, Henderson BE: Estrogens and breast cancer. *Carcinogenesis.*17:2279-2284, 1996.

[14] Bernstein L. The epidemiology of breast cancer. *LOWAC J.* 1:7-13, 1998.

[15] Toniolo PG, Levitz M, Zeleniuch-Jacquotte A, Banerjee S, Koenig KL, Shore RE et al. A prospective study of endogenous estrogens and breast cancer in post-menopausal women. *J. Natl. Cancer Inst.* 86:1076-1082, 1995.

[16] Colditz GA, Hankinson SE, Hunter DJ, Willett EC, Manson JE, Stampfer MJ et al. The use of estrogens and progestins and the risk of breast cancer in postmenopausal women. *N. Engl. J. Med.* 332:1589-1593, 1995.

[17] Key TJA, Pike MC. The dose-effect relationship between "unopposed" estrogens and endometrial mitotic rate: its central role in explaining and predicting endometrial cancer risk. *Br. J. Cancer.* 57:205-212, 1988.

[18] Henderson BE, Ross RK, Pike MC. Hormonal chemoprevention of cancer in women. *Science.*259:633-638, 1993.

[19] Hulka BS, Liu ET, Lininger RA. Steroid hormones and risk of breast cancer. *Cancer.*74:1111-1124, 1993.

[20] Pike M, Bernstein L, Spicer D. Exogenous hormones and breast cancer risk. In: Neiderhuber J (ed). *Current Therapy in Oncol. BC Decker*, St. Louis, MO. pp.292-302, 1993.

[21] Liehr JG. Is estradiol a genotoxic and mutagenic carcinogen? *Endocrine Rev.* 21:40-54, 2000.

[22] Brekelmans CT. Risk factors and risk reduction of breast and ovarian cancer. *Curr. Opin. Obstet. Gynecol.* 15:63-68, 2003.

[23] Bloomgarden ZT. Second World Congress on the Insulin Resistance Syndrome: Mediators, pediatric insulin resistance, the polycystic ovary syndrome, and malignancy. *Diabetes Care.* 28:1821-1830, 2005.

[24] Greenle RT, Murray T, Bolden S, Wongo PA. Cancer statistics. CA *Cancer J. Clin.* 50:7-33, 2000.

[25] Weiderpass E, Gridley G, Persson I et al. Risk of endometrial and breast cancer in patients with diabetes mellitus. *Int. J. Cancer.* 71:360-363, 1997.

[26] Horn LC, Dietel M, Einenkel J. Hormone replacement therapy (HRT) and endometrial morphology under consideration of the different molecular pathways in endometrial carcinogenesis. *Eur. J. Obst. Gyn.Repr. Biol.* 122:4-12, 2005.

[27] Cirisano FD, Robboy SJ, Dodge RK, Bentley RC, Krigman HR, Synan IS, Soper JT, Clarke Pearson DL. The outcome of state I-II clinically and surgically staged papillary serous and clear cell endometrial cancers when compared with endometrial carcinoma. *Gynecol. Oncol.* 77:55-65, 2000.

[28] Siiteri PK, Nisker JA, Hammond GL. Hormonal basis of risk factors for breast and endometrial cancer. In: Iacobelli S, King RJB, Lindner HR, Lippman ME (eds). *Hormones and Cancer*. Raven Press, New York, pp 499-505, 1980.

[29] Greenwald P, Caputo TA, Wolfgang PE. Endometrial cancer after menopausal use of estrogens. *Obstet. Gynecol.* 50:239-243, 1977.

[30] MacMahon B: Risk factors for endometrial cancer. *Gynecol.Oncol.* 2:122-129, 1974.

[31] Key TJ. Hormones and cancer in humans. *Mutat. Res.* 333:59-67, 1995.

[32] La Vecchia C, Franceschi S. Oral contraceptives and ovarian cancer. *Eur.J. Cancer Prev.* 8:297-304, 1999.

[33] Ito K, Utsunomiya H, Yaegashi N, Sasano H. Biological roles of estrogen and progesterone in human endometrial carcinoma – new developments in potential endocrine therapy for endometrial cancer. *Endocrine Journal* 54:667-679, 2007.

[34] Lax SF, Kendall B, Tashiro H, Slebos RJC, Hedrick L. Analysis of p53 and K-ras mutations and microsatellite instability suggests distinct molecular genetic pathways in the pathogenesis of uterine endometrioid and serous carcinoma. *Cancer.* 88:814-824, 2000.

[35] WHO Classification on Pathology and Genetics. In: Tavassoli FA, DevileP(eds): *Tumours of the Breast and Female Genital Organs*. WHO Publications, Geneva, Switzerland. 2003.

[36] Varras M, Polyzos D, Akviris C. Effects of tamoxifen on the human female genital tract: Review of the literature. *Eur. J. Gynaecol. Oncol.* 24:258-268, 2003.

[37] Dietel M, Lewis MA, Shapiro S. Hormone replacement therapy: pathobiological aspects of hormone-sensitive cancers in women relevant to epidemiological studies on HRT: a mini-review. *Human. Reprod.* 20:2052-2060, 2005.

[38] Rodriguez C, Patel AV, Calle EE, Jakob EJ. Estrogen replacement therapy and ovarian cancer mortality in a large prospective study of US women. *J. Am. Med. Assoc.* 285:1460-1465, 2001.

[39] Negri E, Tzonou A, Beral V, Trichopoulos D, Parazzini F, Franceschi S, Booth M, LaVecchia C. Hormonal therapy for menopause and ovarian cancer in a collaborative re-analysis of European studies. *Int. J. Cancer* 80:848-851, 1999.

[40] Lacey JV, Mink PJ, Lubin JH, Sherman ME, Troisi R, Hartge P, Schatzkin A, Schairer C. Menopausal hormone replacement therapy and risk of ovarian cancer. *J. Am. Med. Assoc.*288:334-341, 2002.

[41] Bosetti C, Negri E, Franceschi S, Pelucchi C, Talamini R, Montella M, Conti E, La Vecchia C. Diet and ovarian cancer risk: a case-control study in Italy. *Int. J. Cancer.* 93:911-915, 2001.

[42] International Agency for Research on Cancer: Monographs on the evaluation of carcinogenic risks to humans: hormonal contraception and postmenopausal hormone therapy. IARC, Lyon, France, vol 72, 1999.

[43] Diamanti-Kandarakis E. Hormone replacement therapy and risk of malignancy. *Curr. Opinion Obstet. Gynecol.* 16:73-78, 2004.

[44] Fernandez E, Gallus S, Bosetti C, Franceschi S, Negri E, La Vecchia C. Hormone replacement therapy and cancer risk: a systematic analysis from a network of case-control studies. *Int. J. Cancer.* 105:408-412, 2003.

[45] Ettinger B, Friedman GD, Bush T, Quesenberry CP Jr. Reduced mortality associated with long-term postmenopausal estrogen therapy. *Obstet. Gynecol.* 87:6-12, 1996.

[46] Grodstein F, Clarkson T, Manson J. Understanding the divergent data on postmenopausal hormone therapy. *N. Engl. J. Med.* 348:645-650, 2003.

[47] Gallus S, Bosetti C, Franceschi S, Levi F, Simonato L, Negri E, La Vecchia C. Oesophageal cancer in women: tobacco, alcohol, nutritional and hormonal factors. *Br. J. Cancer.* 85:341-345, 2001.

[48] Olsson H, BladströmAM, Ingvar C. Are smoking-associated cancers prevented or postponed in women using hormone replacement therapy? *Obstet. Gynecol.* 102:565-570, 2003.

[49] Parazzini F, La Vecchia C, Negri E, Franceschi S, Bolis G. Case-control study of estrogen replacement therapy and risk of cervical cancer. *British Med. J.* 315:85-88, 1997.

[50] Rodriguez C, Feigelson HS, Deka A, Patel AV, Jacobs EJ, Thun MJ, Calle EE. Postmenopausal hormone therapy and lung cancer risk in the Cancer Prevention Study II Nutrition Cohort. *Cancer Epidemiol.Biomark. and Prev.* 17:655-660, 2008

[51] Camargo MC, Goto Y, Zabaleta J, Morgan D, Correa P, Rabkin CS. Sex hormones, hormonal interventions and gastric cancer risk: a meta-analysis. *Cancer Epidemiol Biomarkers* Prev Oct 25 [Epub ahead of print] 2011

[52] La Vecchia C, D'Avanzo B, Franceschi S, Negri E, Parazzini F, Decarli A. Menstrual and reproductive factors and gastric-cancer risk in women. *Int. J. Cancer.* 59:761-764, 1994.

[53] Anderson GL, Judd HL, Kaunitz AM et al. Womens's Health Intitative Investigator Effects of estrogen plus progestin on gynaecologic cancers and associated diagnostic producers: The Women's Health Initiative randomised trial. *JAMA.* 290:1739-1748, 2003.

[54] Anderson GL, Limacher M, Assaf AR, Bassford T, Beresford SA, Black H, Bonds D et al. Women's Health Intitative Steering Committee. Effects of conjugated equine estrogen in postmenopausal women with hysterctomy: the Women's Health Intitative randomized controlled trial. *JAMA.*291:1701-1712, 2004.

[55] Hartge P, Harvey EB, Linehan WJ, Silverman DT, Sulivan JW, Hoover RN, Fraumeni JF. Unexplained excess risk of bladder cancer in men. *J.Natl. Cancer Inst.* 82:1636-1640, 1990.

[56] Cantwell MM, Lacey JV Jr, Schairer C, Schatzkin A, Michaud DS. Reproductive factors, exogenous hormone use and bladder cancer risk in a prospective study. *Internat. J. Cancer.* 119:2398-2401, 2006.

[57] McGrath M, Michaud DS, De Vivo I. Hormonal and reproductive factors and the risk of bladder cancer in women. *Am. J. Epidemiol.* 163:236-244,2006.

[58] Gallus S, Bosetti C, Franceschi S, Levi F, Negri E, La Vecchia C. Laryngeal cancer in women. Tobacco, alcohol nutritional and hormonal factors. *Cancer Epidemiol. Biomark. Prev.* 12:512-517, 2003.

[59] Freedman ND, Lacey JV, Hollenbeck AR, Leitzmann MF, Schatzkin A, AbnetChC. The association of menstrual and reproductive factors with upper gastrointestinal tract cancers in the NIH-AARP Cohort. *Cancer.*116:1572-1581, 2010.

[60] Ganti AK, Sahmoun AE, Panwalkar AW, Tendulkar KK, Potti A. Hormone replacement therapy is associated with decreased survival in women with lung cancer. *J. Clin. Oncol.* 24:59-63, 2006.

[61] Kreuzer M, Gerken M, Heinrich J, Kreienbrock L, Wichmann HE. Hormonal factors and risk of lung cancer among women? *Int. J.Epidemiol.*32:263-271, 2003.

[62] Garland CF, Friedlander NJ, Barrett-Conner E, Khaw KT. Sex hormones and postmenopausal breast cancer: a prospective study in an adult community. *Am. J. Epidemiol.* 135:1220-1230, 1992.

[63] Wysowski KK, Comstock GW, Helsing KJ, Lau HL. Sex hormone levels in serum in relation to the development of breast cancer. *Am. J.Epidemiol.* 125:791-799, 1987.

[64] Stefanick ML, Anderson GL, Margolis KL, Hendrix SJ et al. Effects of conjugated equine estrogens on breast cancer and mammography screening in postmenopausal women with hysterectomy. *JAMA.*295:1647-1657, 2006.

[65] LaCroix AZ, Chlebowski RT, Manson JE, Aragaki AK, Johnson KC, Martin L et al. Health outcomes after stopping conjugated equine estrogens among postmenopausal women with prior hysterectomy. A randomized controlled trial. *JAMA.* 305:1305-1314, 2011.

[66] Anderson GL, Chlebowski RT, Aragaki AK, Kuller LH, Manson JE, Gass M, Bluhm E, Connelly S, Hubbell FA, Lane D, Martin L, Ockene J, Rohan T, Schenken R, Wactawski-Wende J. Conjugated equine oestrogen and breast cancer incidence and mortality in postmenopausal women with hysterectomy: extended follow-up of the Women's Health Initiative randomised placebo-controlled trial. *Lancet Oncol.* 2012 Mar 6. [Epub ahead of print].

[67] Hulley S, Grady D, Busch T et al. Randomized trial of estrogen plus progestin for secondary prevention of coronary heart disease in postmenopausal women: heart and Estrogen/Progestin Replacement Study (Hers) Research Group. *JAMA.* 380:605-613, 1998.

[68] Risch HA. Hormone replacement therapy and the risk of ovarian cancer. *Gynecol.Oncol.* 86:115-117, 2002.

[69] Shapiro S. False alarm: postmenopausal hormone therapy and ovarian cancer. *Climacteric.* 10:466-470, 2007.

[70] Grady D. Postmenopausal hormones – therapy for symptoms only. *NewEngl. J. Med.* 348:1-3, 2003.

[71] Collaborative Group on Hormonal Factors in Breast Cancer. Collaborative reanalysis of data from 51 epidemiological studies of 52 705 women with breast cancer and 108 411 women without breast cancer. *Lancet.* 350:1047-1059, 1997.

[72] Adami HO, Signorello LB, and Trichopolos D. Towards an understanding of breast cancer etiology. *Semin. Cancer Biol.* 8:255-262, 1998.

[73] Hofseth LJ, RaafatAM, Osuch JR, Pathak DR, Slomski CA, Haslam SZ. Hormone replacement therapy with estrogen or estrogen plus medroxy-progesterone acetate is associated with increased epithelial proliferation in the normal postmenopausal breast. *J. Clin. Endocrinol. Metab.* 84:4559-4565, 1999.

[74] Li CI, Weiss NS, Stanford JL, Daling JR. Hormone replacement therapy in relation to risk of lobular and ductal breast carcinoma in middle-aged women. *Cancer*.88:2570-2577, 2000.

[75] Wisemann RA. Breast cancer hypothesis: a single cause for the majority of cases. *J. Epidemiol. Community Health.* 54:851-858, 2000.

[76] Spratt JS, Meyer JS, Spratt JA. Rates of growth of human solid neoplasms: part I. *J. Surg. Oncol.* 60:137-146, 1995.

[77] Shackney SE, McCormack GW, JrCuchural GJ. Growth rate patterns of solid tumors and their relation to responsiveness to therapy: an analytical review. *Ann Intern Med.* 89:107-121, 1978.

[78] Spratt JS, Spratt JA. What is breast cancer doing before we can detect it? *J. Surg. Oncol.* 1985;30:156-160.

[79] Haskell CM. Thorax. Unknown primary-breast cancer in cancer treatment, 2nd ed. WB Saunders Company, 1985.

[80] Anderson TJ, Battersby S, King RJB et al. Oral contraceptive use influences resting breast proliferation. *Hum. Pathol.* 20:1139-1144, 1989.

[81] SubaZs. Estrogen deficiency as cancer risk factor. Chapter 5. In: *Estrogen versus cancer*. Nova Science Publishers, Inc. New York, 2009.

[82] SubaZs. Systemic risk factors for oral cancer: Estrogen deficiency and insulin resistance. Chapter 8. pp: 157-172 In: *Progress in Oral Cancer Research.* Ed: Frederik L. Nielsen, Nova Science Publishers, New York, 2008.

[83] Coulam CB, Annegers JF, Kranz JS. Chronic anovulation syndrome and associated neoplasia. *Obstet. Gynecol.* 61:403-407, 1983.

[84] Hartge P. Abortion, breast cancer and epidemiology. *N. Engl. J. Med.* 336:127-128, 1997.

[85] Pierpoint T, McKeigue PM, Isaacs AJ, Wild SH, Jacobs HS. Mortality of women with polycystic ovary syndrome at long-term follow-up. *J.Clin. Epidemiol.* 51:581-586,1998.

[86] Gadducci A, Gargini A, Palla E, Fanucchi A, Genazzani AR. Polycystic ovary syndrome and gynecological cancers: is there a link? *Gynecol.Endocrinol.* 20:200-208, 2005.

[87] Sartor BM, Dickey RP. Polycystic ovarian syndrome and the metabolic syndrome. *Am. J. Med.* 330:336-342, 2005.

[88] Spritzer PM, Morsch DM, Wiltgen D. Polycystic ovary syndrome associated neoplasms. *Arq. Bras. Endocrinol. Metabol.* 49:805-810, 2006.

[89] Nestler JE, Strauss JF. Insulin as an effector of human ovarian and adrenal steroid metabolism. *Endocrin. Metab. Clin. North. Amer.* 20:807-823, 1991.

[90] Polson DW, Wadsworth J, Adams J et al. Polycystic ovaries: a common finding in normal women. *Lancet.* 1:870-872, 1988.

[91] Carmina E, Lobo RA. Polycystic ovaries in hirsute women with normal menses. *Am. J. Med.* 111:602-606, 2001.

[92] Farquhar CM, Birdsall M, Manning P et al. The prevalence of polycystic ovaries on ultrasound scanning in a population of randomly selected women. *Aust. NZ. Obstet.Gynaecol.* 34:67-72, 1994.

[93] Llewellyn CD, Johnson NW, Warnakulasuriya KAAS. Risk factors for squamous cell carcinoma of the oral cavity in young people-a comprehensive literature review. *Oral Oncol.* 37:401-418, 2001.

[94] Björnström L, Sjöberg M. Mechanisms of estrogen receptor signaling: Convergence of genomic and nongenomic actions on target genes. *Molecular Endocrinol.* 19:833-842, 2005.

[95] Pillay OC, Te Fong LF, Crow JC, Benjamin E, Mould T, Atiomo W, Menon PA, Leonard AJ, Hardiman P. The association between polycystic ovaries and endometrial cancer. *Human Reprod.* 21:924-929, 2006.

[96] Miller WR, O'Neill J. The importance of local synthesis of estrogen within the breast. *Steroids.* 50:537-548, 1987.

[97] Santen RJ, Martel J, Hoagland M, Naftolin F, Roa L, Harada N, Hafer L, Zaino R, Santner SJ. Stromal spindle cells contain aromatase in human breast-tumors. *J. Clin. Endocrin.Metab.* 79:627-632, 1994.

[98] McCullough LD, Blizzard K, Simpson ER, Öz OK, Hurn PD. Aromatase cytochrome P450 and extragonadal estrogen play a role in ischemic neuroprotection. *J. Neurosci.* 23:8701-8705, 2003.

[99] Faustini-Fustini M, Rochira V, Carani C. Oestrogen deficiency in men: where are we today? *Eur. J. Endocrinol.* 140:111-129, 1999.

[100] Carani C, Qin K, Simoni M, Faustini-Fustini M, Serpente S, Boyd J et al. Effect of testosterone and estradiol a in man with aromatase deficiency. *New Engl. J. Med.* 337:91-95, 1997.

[101] Smith EP, Boyd J, Frank GR, Takahashi H, Cohen RM, Specker B et al. Estrogen resistance caused by a mutation in the estrogen receptor gene in a man. *New Engl. J. Med.* 331:1056-1061, 1994.

In: Estrogen Prevention for Breast Cancer
Editor: Zsuzsanna Suba

ISBN: 978-1-62417-378-3

Chapter II

Interaction between Insulin and Estrogen in the Regulation of Cell Proliferation and Carcinogenesis

Zsuzsanna Suba
National Institute of Oncology, Department of Surgical and Molecular Pathology, Budapest, Hungary

Abstract

Both insulin resistance and estrogen deficiency result in complex metabolic disorder based mainly on the defective cellular glucose uptake and on an atherogenic serum lipid profile. These alterations may be regarded as high risks for several life-threatening human diseases, such as type-2 diabetes, cardiovascular lesions and malignancies. Insulin resistance and estrogen deficiency are concomitant disorders with mutual interrelationship. Insulin resistance and the compensatory hyperinsulinemia provoke increased androgen synthesis at the expense of decreased estrogen production. Similarly, a moderate or severe decrease in serum estrogen levels enhances the prevalence of insulin resistant states both in men and women. Healthy premenopausal women enjoy the defensive effect of estrogens against metabolic and hormonal disorders. However, even a slight decrease in their circulatory estrogen levels associated with insulin resistance may increase the risk for cancers, particularly in the organs having high estrogen demand (breast, endometrium and ovary). On the other hand, postmenopausal state with profound estrogen deficiency confers high risk for cancers in different organs with either high or moderate estrogen demand. After menopause, hormone replacement therapy improves insulin sensitivity and decreases the enhanced inclination to malignancies in postmenopausal women.

Recognition of thorough interplay between insulin resistance and estrogen deficiency may illuminate many apparently controversial experimental and clinical findings concerning cancer development and therapeutic possibilities. Moreover, their interactions in the initiation and progression of human malignancies may supply new strategies in the primary cancer prevention and cancer cure.

Introduction

Insulin has pivotal roles in the facilitation of anabolic processes and in the activation of transport systems being associated with the metabolism of carbohydrates proteins and lipids [1]. It is also a potent regulator of human sexual steroid hormone synthesis and interferes with their signal transduction at cellular level. Insulin resistance is a disorder of cellular glucose uptake and results in a complex metabolic and hormonal disturbance [2]. It may be regarded as high risk for several life-threatening human diseases, such as type-2 diabetes, cardio-vascular lesions and malignancies [3].

Actions of female sexual steroids are much wider than having crucial roles in female physiology and reproduction. Estrogen receptor signals are fairly involved in the beneficial regulation of metabolic processes and in the gene regulation of cell growth, differentiation and proliferation both in men and women [4].Physiological estrogen levels in healthy premenopausal women supply a favor against hypertension and cardiovascular diseases as compared with men in the same age. However, after menopause a decreased ovarian estrogen synthesis will be associated with a rapidly increasing prevalence of ischemic stroke, myocardial infarction and pulmonary emboli among women [5].

Both insulin and estrogens transfer potent mitogenic stimuli and share important functions in the control of cell proliferation. This suggests that an equilibrium of their signal transduction pathways have crucial role in cancer prevention.

Insulin resistance and estrogen deficiency are concordant disorders and they have mutual interrelationship [6]. Moderate or severe estrogen deficiency proved to be a high risk factor for insulin resistance both in premenopausal and postmenopausal women as well as in male cases [7,8,9,10]. On the other hand insulin resistance and hyperinsulinemia provoke a severe imbalance in the sexual steroid synthesis resulting in excessive androgen and low estrogen levels and interferes with estrogen effect even at receptor level [11].

Our knowledge concerning the consequences of insulin resistance is relatively young; its multifaceted metabolic and vascular complications were revealed near the end of the 20th century [12]. Recognition of correlations between insulin resistance and malignancies suffered several years' delay, but recently the role of insulin resistance in the initiation and progression of cancer has been undoubtedly justified [13]. On the contrary, estrogen deficiency had been a traditional etiologic factor for postmenopausal cardiovascular diseases and stroke for a long time, however, its correlation with cancer risk remained obscure till now.

The currently prevailing concept is the carcinogenic capacity of estrogen, especially for the highly estrogen responsive organs of women. The Women's Health Initiative (WHI) hormone replacement therapy trial included more than 161 000 women and worked on strategies for the prevention of heart disease, bone fracture and breast cancer in postmenopausal women. Results of this study as originally interpreted established that estrogen treatment was associated with a high incidence of breast cancer [14].

Estrogen deficiency as a cancer risk factor emerged first in a study on Hungarian oral cancer cases in 2007 [15]. Accumulation of non-smoker, non-drinker elderly postmenopausal female cases among oral cancer patients suggested a heretical idea: carcinogenic capacity of estrogen deficiency. This newly revealed correlation means a contradiction to the traditional concept of estrogen-induced breast cancer.Critical reevaluation of the contradictory results of hormone replacement therapy yielded a complete conversion: no estrogen but rather its deficiency may cause cancer initiation [16].

Recently a sensational review and reanalysis reversed the earlier results of WHI hormone replacement therapy trial. The authors established that estrogen is not carcinogenic rather a protective agent for breast cancer risk, as well as for many other aspects of women's health [17]. This shocking result may help after a long delay to focus on estrogen deficiency as cancer risk factor.

The present study gives a short review on the proven carcinogenic capacity of insulin resistance and a balanced analysis of the controversial epidemiologic and experimental associations between estradiol and cancer risk. As a further step, this work summarizes the mutual correlations between insulin resistance and estrogen deficiency as players in cancer development.

Correlations between Insulin Resistance and Cancer Risk

Insulin resistance (IR) is a defect of insulin-mediated cellular glucose uptake, which may elicit many disorders in the gene regulation of cellular metabolism, growth, differentiation and mitotic activity [13].

Discovery of IR as a complex metabolic disturbance was a milestone in understanding the base of human illnesses [2]. Nowadays, IR is regarded as a worldwide risk factor for the two most dangerous human disease groups; namely for arteriosclerotic cardiovascular lesions and malignancies [13]. Insulin resistance syndrome has five basic criteria: hyperglycemia, visceral obesity, elevated serum triglyceride and low HDL-cholesterol level (dyslipidemia) and hypertension. Each of these criteria alone is cancer risk factor and they mean together a multiple risk [3].

The first, compensated phase of insulin resistance in the liver, skeletal muscles and fatty tissue leads to reactive hyperinsulinemia by the increased secretory capacity of the insular β-cells and the serum glucose level remains within the normal range. Insulin has diverse metabolic effects and at the same time functions as a growth factor and the elevation of insulin level in itself is a high cancer risk [18]. Hyperinsulinemia increases the production and mitogenic activity of other, insulin-like growth factors, such as IGF-I and IGF-II, which have important role in the cell proliferation and tumor induction at several sites [19].

In the second uncompensated phase of insulin resistance the secretor capacity of insular β-cells is exhausted and with elevation of fasting glucose (EFG) type-2 diabetes develops. Hyperglycemia promotes the increased DNA-synthesis of tumor cells by several pathways [20]. It provokes excessive deliberation of free radicals, which will cause the derangement of both DNA and enzymes having role in the repair mechanisms and leads to harmful non-enzymatic glycation of protein structures.

All phases of IR are proven risk factors for pancreas, liver, colon, urinary bladder, prostate, salivary gland and oral cavity cancers and even for the malignancies of the highly estrogen responsive breast, ovary and endometrium [15, 20-29]. Nowadays we are on the route to regard malignancies as complications of IR. Tumor progression is promoted by IR as well. In cancer patients with EFG or type-2 diabetes the rate of tumor recurrence, metastatic spread and fatal outcome is higher as compared with patients without metabolic disease [3].

Recognition of correlations between IR and tumor development reveals new possibilities in primary and secondary cancer prevention. Healthy diet, physical activity and weight loss increase insulin sensitivity and decrease the risk for both cardiovascular diseases and malignancies.

Historical Review of Associations between Estrogen and Cancer Development

Epidemiological Data Suggesting the Carcinogenic Capacity of Estrogen

Idea of correlation between female sexual steroids and breast cancer risk had emerged more than 100 years ago [30]. From the early 1980s epidemiological and clinical studies have increasingly pointed to an elevated breast, endometrial and ovarian cancer risk associated with estrogens [31,32,33,34,35,36].

Even a slightly elevated serum level of endogenous estrogen was regarded as risk for breast cancer [27,33,37]. Exogenous estrogens alone or in combination with progestin were found also to be risk factors for breast cancer [34,36,38,39]. Pike et al. summarized the results of population based epidemiological studies that had been published supporting the relative breast cancer risk from the use of postmenopausal hormone replacement therapy (HRT) [40]. Available literary data suggested that the use of HRT for more than 5-10 years means an increased relative risk for breast cancer [41].

Hyperestrogenism is regarded as a causal factor for endometrial hyperplasia and later to epithelial atypia, which may be the predecessor of endometrial adenocarcinoma. Epidemiologists accepted exogenous estrogen administration as a risk factor for human endometrial carcinoma [42].

In the USA an increased risk of ovarian cancer mortality was associated with postmenopausal estrogen use based on a large prospective study [43]. A collaborative reanalysis of European studies found a relative risk of ovarian cancer for ever use of HRT [44]. Recently, in a cohort study a strong relationship was established between the duration of estrogen therapy and risk of ovarian cancer [45].

Carcinogenic activity of steroidal estrogens has been summarized in 2000 by the International Agency for Research on Cancer (IARC), which classified the evidences for these effects in humans [46].

Controversies of Experimental Results Concerning the Carcinogenic Capacity of Estrogen

Though earlier epidemiological studies have long been suspected that estrogens play a central role in breast cancer development, the mechanism of their carcinogenic capacity on human breast epithelial cells has not yet been clearly demonstrated [47].

Hormonal contribution of estrogen to carcinogenesis is based on its physiological functions in gene regulation [48]. Estrogen-induced proliferation of human tumor cell line and renal carcinogenesis induced by excessive estrogen doses in Syrian hamsters were inhibited by hormone antagonists [49]. These results were evaluated as crucial role of estrogen receptors in tumor growth either by fixation of spontaneous mutations or by induction of DNA damages. However, in these models only the excessive overdosage of estrogen could induce tumors, which has no predicting value in carcinogen testing [50]. Bacterial and mammalian gene mutation assays failed to justify any *mutagenic activity of estrogen* [51,52].

Epigenetic, estrogen-induced carcinogenesis was also proposed via estrogen receptor-mediated proliferation of mammary epithelial cells carrying spontaneous replication errors [33]. However, the absence of ERs in proliferating human mammary epithelial cells provided evidence against this assumed carcinogenic pathway [53].

Carcinogenesis by covalent modification of estrogen receptors was also a proposed mechanism and through this route a permanent stimulation of receptors was suggested to induce uncontrolled cell proliferation [54]. However, further studies could not justify the estrogen-induced carcinogenesis by covalent receptor modification [55]. *Catechol metabolites ofestrogen* were demonstrated to induce neoplastic transformation in human endometrial cells [56]. However, the rate of catecholestrogen production proved to be too low to result in significant amounts of genotoxic metabolites [51].

Estrogen-induced chromosomal abnormalities emerged also as explanation for carcinogenic capacity. Chromosomal changes or genome mutations might be provoked by estrogen in cell cultures and in laboratory animals [57,58]. However, the estrogen induced neoplastic transformation of Syrian hamster embryo cells was reported without detectable concomitant gene mutations [59]. These results suggested that in addition to spontaneous chromosomal abnormalities other mutations are necessary for cells to acquire carcinogenic capacity.

Free radical mediated DNA-damage also emerged as an indirect mechanism of estrogen-induced carcinogenesis. Concentrations of 8-hydroxyguanine DNA bases, formed by hydroxy radical reaction, were increased in DNA incubated by catecholestrogens [60]. However, literary data has established that estrogens have definite antioxidant activity and protective effect against oxidative stress especially in premenopausal women [61].

In vitro experiments, which tried to clarify the carcinogenic mechanism of estrogen effect, were fairly simplified models disregarding the cross talks and feedback mechanisms of mediators under biological circumstances.

Recent Results Supporting the Anticancer Capacity of Estrogen

Differences in exposure to known exogenous risk factors in men and women don't seem to explain the sex differences in cancer incidence rates. Recently, the justified associations of healthy reproductive and menstrual factors with decreased cancer risk in women helped to explain their lower tumor incidence rate as compared with men [15,62].

Later menopause and *longer duration of fertile life* in women seemed to be inversely associated with the risk for cancers of urinary bladder, stomach, oral cavity and upper gastrointestinal tract [15,62,63,64]. Vast majority of authors supposed that female sexual steroids help to maintain the local integrity of epithelial surfaces, which may counteract exogenous carcinogenic agents. Nevertheless, estrogen may also exert a systemic anticancer capacity by its advantageous effects on hormonal, metabolic and immunologic processes [16].

Many studies have found an inverse relationship between *parity and cancer risk*; concerning breast, endometrial, urinary bladder, pancreas and oral cancers [65,66,67,68]. It remained unclear how parity may decrease the cancer risk but presumably, a healthy equilibrium of female sexual steroid production associated with good fertility may have tumor protective impact at several sites [69].

Hormone replacement therapy (HRT) in postmenopausal women supplies excellent possibilities to study the associations between female sexual steroid hormones and tumor incidence. Till now, the prevailing concept is that HRT is associated with an increased prevalence of gynecological and breast cancers [32,35].

By contrast, recent clinical studies on HRT user women yielded beneficial anticancer effects against oral, esophageal, gastric, colorectal, cervical, liver and lung cancers [32,64,70,71,72,73,74]. Moreover, a decreased risk for endometrial cancer could also be observed among postmenopausal women with HRT use [75]. Doubts concerning associations between estrogen treatment and ovarian cancer risk have also emerged [76]. These results suggest a systemic protective effect of estrogen against cancers at several sites.

Nowadays, breast cancer remained as a last fortress to support the principle of the carcinogenic capacity of estrogen. However, in 2004, in the WHI Randomized Controlled Trial, the estrogen treatment of women with prior hysterectomy over 6-8 years reduced significantly the breast cancer risk [77]. The authors suggested further investigations to justify this unexpected result. Recently, in 2011, a continued follow up study of the same trial on hysterectomized cases strengthened a significantly lower risk for breast cancer in estrogen-treated survivor women [78]. Considering the principle of estrogen deficiency induced cancer, the breast cancer risk of women after hysterectomy may be near uniformly high. Their abrupt, shocking hormone deprivation may be more dangerous for the health as compared with those undergoing natural menopause. HRT studies on these homogenously selected cases seem to be much more reliable [16].

A sensational study was published in 2010, which re-evaluated the earlier results of WHI Hormone Replacement Therapy Trial suggesting a strong carcinogenic capacity of estrogen for the female breast [14]. After a proper selection of the same cases HRT use proved to be not only safe but rather protective for breast cancer risk [17]. This conversion is not surprising if we take into consideration that breast cancer is a multicausal disease and the previous WHI study examined the involved women in two pooled groups; cases with and without hormone treatment. WHI authors disregarded the individual reproductive and menstrual differences and other known or suspected risk factors for breast cancer and the obtained results were misleading [16]. These recent, methodologically correct examinations yielded excellent proofs for the protective effect of estrogen even for breast cancer risk. The walls of the last fortress seem to be crumbling.

Ambiguous Functions of Estrogen in the Regulation of Cell Proliferation

Estrogen receptors (ERs) belong to the steroid-thyroid hormone nuclear receptor superfamily [79]. The classic, genomic mechanism of ER action is that estrogen binding activates Ers in the nucleus and they act as transcriptional modulators by binding to specific sequences in the promoter region of target genes [4,80]. Ers can also regulate gene expression without direct binding to DNA by interaction with transcription factor proteins, which may result in either stimulation or inhibition in gene transcription processes [79]. Moreover, Ers may regulate the expression of genes that do not contain estrogen responsive elements (EREs).

Estrogen have also non-genomic actions by membrane-associated ER signaling cascades, which may influence both the functions of cytoplasmic protein network and the regulation of gene expression in the nucleus [81]. Finally, genomic and non-genomic pathways of ER signaling converge on the target genes [4]. This complex signaling system provides an exquisitely safety control and plasticity of tissue responses to estrogen modified by the nature of temporary intra- and extracellular stimuli.

There are two receptor isoforms; ER-α and ER-β, which are widely expressed throughout the body with a predominance of one or the other [79]. Both ER isoforms are markedly expressed in the mammary glands, uterus, brain, bone and cardiovascular system. All these sites are especially endangered in postmenopausal women by the decreased hormone production of ovaries. Ischemic attacks in the central nervous system, osteoporosis and cardiovascular diseases show conspicuously increased prevalence in women after menopause. Cancer risk of moderate estrogen loss in young women, especially in the highly estrogen responsive organs; such as breast, endometrium and ovary seems to be a newly recognized danger [16].

Estrogen receptor isoforms (ER-α and ER-β) differently regulate the cell proliferation and apoptotic cell death. In a mammary gland epithelial cell line, deriving from pregnant mouse, selective agonists for ER-α provoked cell proliferation, whereas agonists for ER-β induced inhibitory effect [82]. Mouse mammary cell line could exhibit physiological resistance to estradiol induced cell proliferation as concomitant activation of ER isoforms may equalize the opposing cellular responses.

Embryonic development well demonstrates the physiologic role of all the ambiguous actions of estrogen [83]. High estrogen levels in pregnant women might ensure explosion-like cell proliferation in the developing embryonic tissues and organs due to the predominance of ERα signaling pathways. By contrast, when the growth should be stopped, cessation of high mitotic activity results in a dynamic equilibrium of cell number conducted by a concomitant activation of both receptor isoforms. Moreover, by the predominance of ER-β activity, a stimulation of apoptotic cell death may induce an involution of embryonic structures, which have lost their function.

Crosstalk between ER and GFR (growth factor receptor) signaling pathways are well-known both in healthy tissues and malignancies. Estradiol liganded ERs in the plasma membrane can rapidly transactivate the epidermal growth factor receptor (EGFR) or insulin-like growth factor-I receptor (IGF-IR) by feedback mechanism [84]. Estradiol may induce both growth stimulation and growth inhibition depending on the ratio and activity of ERs and GFRs [85]. On the other hand, the mitogen associated protein kinase (MAPK) system of GFR signaling is capable to modulate the aminoterminal activity of ERs by phosphorylation [86].

In human breast cancer cells, expressions of ERs and EGFRs are often inversely correlated [87]. Inhibition of growth factor signaling in apparently ER-negative breast cancer cells successfully restored ER expression suggesting a dynamic, inverse relationship between the two receptor systems [88]. Estrogen treatment could inhibit lung carcinogenesis by the reduction of IGF-I level, which is a potent mitogenic agent for malignancies [89]. These results suggest rather an alternative role of estrogen and growth factor actions in tumor cell proliferation. Nevertheless, the presumed synergistic contribution of ERs and GFRs to cancer development and progression would be a permanent danger without contraregulatory impact.

In emergency situation of estrogen deficiency, GF initiated activities may induce estradiol specific ER responses by a physiological coupling of the two signaling pathways when intact nuclear ERs are available [90,91]. However, a permanent absence of estrogen may induce overwhelming GF signals. Unopposed GF signaling may modulate the functions of exposed, non-liganded ERs through the phosphorylation of certain receptor residues [85]. Predominance of GF activities and an alteration of non-liganded ERs may provoke a breakdown in the gene regulation of cell proliferation beyond retrieval [16,69].

Molecular Mechanism of Interplay between the Actions of Estrogen and Insulin

Effects of Estrogen on Glucose Metabolism

Estrogen has beneficial effects on the energy metabolism and glucose homeostasis by means of several possible pathways [92]. It regulates the insulin production capacity of the pancreatic islet cells [93]. In the liver, estrogen regulates insulin sensitivity by the activation of glycogen synthetase and glycolytic enzymes and advantageously modulates the glucose uptake of peripheral target tissues as well [94,95]. Experimental and clinical studies justify that estrogen deficiency or alterations in ER signal transduction result in insulin resistance.

Increased insulin secretion of pancreatic β-cells controls elevated plasma glucose level during the post-prandial phase. In animal experiments ovarectomy is associated with an increased risk of diabetes, whereas estrogen treatment improves the insulin response to glucose load [96]. Estrogen administration enhanced the glucose-induced insulin secretion in rat pancreas and in mouse islet cells [93]. These data might explain the suppression of glucose induced insulin secretion in estrogen deficiency.

In aromatase knockout (ArKO) mice the enzyme for estrogen biosynthesis is inactivated, and these estrogen deficient animals are insulin resistant; they have reduced glucose oxidation, increased adiposity and high insulin levels. Glucose intolerance of ArKO mice can be reversed by estrogen treatment both in females and males [97]!.

After menopause, type-2 diabetes and obesity may be only partially reversed by restricted diet because it cannot improve pancreatic β-cell mass and function. However, in postmenopausal women regular physical activity or estrogen replacement alone has more beneficial antidiabetogenic effect suggesting their direct improving impact on the insulin secretion capacity of β-cells [93].

In the liver, insulin regulates the glucose uptake and glucose output and ensures glucose homeostasis in case of normal insulin sensitivity [92]. Estrogen receptors have crucial roles in the glucose metabolism of the liver. In ER-α receptor knockout (ERKO) animals, hepatic insulin resistance is associated with decreased glucose uptake in the skeletal muscles [94]. These findings reveal that estrogen receptor-alpha plays an important role in the regulation of glucose homeostasis and of insulin sensitivity in mice.

Estrogen receptors are newly recognized important players in glucose metabolism [92]. They advantageously modulate insulin stimulated cellular glucose uptake through the regulation of the tyrosine phosphorylation of insulin receptor protein [98].

ERs have crucial roles in cellular glucose uptake by the regulation of glucose transporter (GLUT) containing cytoplasmic vesicles. They participate both in GLUT4 expression and translocation. In ovarectomized rats, estradiol substitution increased the amount of GLUT1 protein in the blood-brain barrier [99].In immature rat uterus estradiol treatment caused a fourfold increase in GLUT1 protein content and also increased glucose uptake [95]. In polycystic ovarium syndrome (PCOS) cases, in which an ovarian overproduction of testosterone is characteristic, insulin stimulated glucose uptake was reduced due to decreased amounts of GLUT4 on adipocyte membrane [100].

ER-α and ER-β seem to have opposite actions on glucose homeostasis and modulation of GLUT4 activities. Mice that lack ER-α are insulin resistant; exhibit impaired glucose tolerance and obesity, affecting both males and females. By contrast, ER-β activation might have a diabetogenic effect and opposes the action of ER-α [92]. Presumably, a continuously adjusted balance between ER-α and ER-β maintains the ideal GLUT4 expression and glucose homeostasis.

Higher concentrations of estradiol can inhibit insulin signaling by modulation of insulin receptor substrate-1 (IRS-l) phosphorylation in adipocytes [101]. As insulin has not only metabolic but also mitogenic effects, an inhibition of excessive insulin receptor signal by estrogen may be a safety impact both against pathological glucose uptake and cell proliferation.

Estrogens have pivotal role in growth hormone (GH) activity by means of inhibitory or stimulatory effects on its secretion and on cellular GH receptor functions. These observations suggest that estrogens play a major and positive role in the regulation of GH-IGF-I axis in both genders [102], which may be in close correlation with their antidiabetogenic and anticancer capacities.

Effects of Estrogen on Lipid Metabolism and Fat Deposition

Estrogen has positive regulatory effects on the maintenance of serum lipid levels, on the insulin sensitivity of adipocytes and on advantageous body fat distribution. Postmenopausal women exhibit more atherogenic serum lipid profile as compared with premenopausal cases and estrogen treatment may reduce the risk of cardiovascular disease by favorable changes in plasma lipid levels [103].

In aged rats, estradiol administration lowered the level of lipid peroxidation and improved the dysfunction parameters of the liver [104]. Moreover, an androgen receptor-mediated antagonism of estrogen-dependent low-density lipoprotein receptor (LDLR) transcription was observed in cultured hepatocytes [105]. This observation may partially reveal the antagonistic associations of male and female sexual steroids with lipid metabolism and vascular diseases.

Estrogen regulates the total mass, regional body distribution and metabolism of adipose tissue, which plays a pivotal role in energy homeostasis, insulin sensitivity and immune responses [106].

In healthy premenopausal women central, abdominal adipocytes show higher insulin sensitivity than in male cases [107], which means lower risk for insulin resistance in the generative period of women. However, menopause results in increased central adiposity and higher fasting insulin levels suggesting higher risk for metabolic and cardiovascular diseases [93,108] and for malignancies [109].

Obesity is an excessive deposition of adipose tissue and predisposes patients to a variety of diseases such as; cardiovascular lesions, type-2 diabetes and malignancies [110]. Obesity and overweight are important concomitants of insulin resistance and disturbed equilibrium of male to female sexual hormone concentrations in women [111]. There are controversial correlations between increased body weight and estrogen action. Some authors could find linear correlation between high body mass index (BMI) and elevated serum estrogen level [110]. Others observed associations between androgen excess and central adiposity both in pre- and postmenopausal cases [112].

There are major sex differences in insulin sensitivity and the deposition of adipose tissue. Estrogens induce predominantly gluteofemoral adipose tissue deposition, whereas in case of androgen excess rather intraabdominal fat accumulation is typical [108]. "Android women" with excessive circulatory androgen levels exhibit central obesity, which is strongly associated with insulin resistance and its complications [111,112].

Effects of Insulin on Sexual Steroid Hormone Production and on Their Signals at Receptor Level

Insulin is a potent effector of human sexual steroid hormone production in the endocrine organs and modulates estrogen signals at receptor level as well.

In women insulin resistance may contribute to hyperandrogenism and anovulatory dysfunction through several pathways [113]. Hyperinsulinemia in the first, compensated phase of insulin resistance stimulates the testosterone biosynthesis of human ovarian theca cells from women with polycystic ovarian syndrome (PCOS) [114]. This results in excessive androgen and deficient estrogen production. Treatment by insulin sensitizing Metformin reduced the hyperinsulinemia and inhibited directly the androgen overproduction in human ovarian theca cells [115].

Insulin may affect the pituitary to favor the secretion of luteinizing hormone (LH) and increases adrenal androgen production by means of an increased adrenal sensitivity to adrenocorticotropin [116].Insulin and insulin-like growth factor-I receptors may synergize with LH to promote androgen production by ovarian theca cells [114].

There are contradictions concerning the hormonal and metabolic disturbances in PCOS cases and the interpretation of complications in such patients. High risk for endometrial cancer in women with PCOS was presumed to justify the "unopposed estrogen hypothesis" supposing normal or elevated bioavailable estrogen, but low level of progesterone [36].Nevertheless, both obesity and hyperinsulinemia in these cases are associated with defective ovarian estrogen and excessive androgen synthesis [11], thus unopposed high estrogen level cannot be blamed for endometrial cancer risk. Moreover, high estrogen level would be contradictory to anovulatory infertility as ovulation may be provoked by excessive estrogen administration.Recently, androgen-excess and the associated metabolic alterations are regarded as common sources of cardiovascular risk and other complications in PCOS cases [117]. Hyperandrogenism explains both anovulation and hirsutism, which are characteristic disorders in women with PCOS.

Clinical Correlations between Estrogen Deficiency, Insulin Resistance and Cancer Risk

A moderate or severe decrease in female sexual steroid hormone levels enhances the prevalence of insulin resistant states both in premenopausal and postmenopausal cases. On the other hand, elevated fasting glucose, type-2 diabetes and obesity are closely associated with anovulation and altered reproductive functions in young women and with postmenopausal changes in the elderly [9,10].

In premenopausal women long or highly irregular menstrual cycles suggesting defective ovarian function are predictors for risk of type-2 diabetes [118]. In young women endometrial cancer risk shows close correlation with nulliparity, irregular menstrual cycles, diabetes and hypertension [28]. In conclusion, the hormonal treatment of menstrual disorders helps to lower the risk for both diabetes and endometrial cancer.

Polycystic ovarium syndrome (PCOS) in young women is an important pathologic example of correlations between the disturbed equilibrium of sexual steroids and insulin resistance [13]. The cardinal symptoms are anovulation, infertility, hirsutism and obesity. In PCOS cases insulin resistance and hyperinsulinemia overregulate ovarian androgen synthesis at the expense of decreased estrogen production. Use of insulin sensitizing drugs in PCOS cases lowered serum insulin level and improved menstrual abnormalities, ovulatory dysfunction, infertility and hirsutism [11].

Insulin resistance in PCOS cases means general health risk for the affected women. Metabolic syndrome and type-2 diabetes has been shown to be consistently frequent among women with PCOS diagnosis [9,119]. Moreover, an increased prevalence of premature cardiovascular diseases and malignancies, preferentially in breast, endometrium and ovaries were observed in PCOS cases [117,120]. In a mortality study on patients with PCOS breast cancer proved to be the leading cause of death [121].

In "android women" the excessive androgen level may be due to the decreased conversion of testosterone to estrogen by aromatase cytochrome P450, resulting in decreased estrogen level [111]. Hyperandrogenism in women is closely associated with insulin resistance and disorders of fertility. These patients have male characteristics of muscle mass, visceral adiposity and increased risk of hypertension, type-2 diabetes and cardiovascular disease [112,117,122]. Visceral obesity and type-2 diabetes are in close correlation with tumor development.

In the *climacteric and postmenopausal period*, the increased body weight and central obesity are often observed in women and the prevalence of metabolic syndrome and type-2 diabetes increase dramatically with age [123,124,125,126,127]. Theories emerged that estrogen deficiency and increased androgen activity are responsible for the worsening of glucose homeostasis in postmenopausal women [128].

Cancer risk shows strong correlations with elevated fasting glucose level, hyperinsulinemia, increased IGF level, hypertriglyceridemia, type-2 diabetes and excessive body weight [20,110,124,125]. These alterations are more frequent among postmenopausal women as compared with younger cases. In postmenopausal women a progressive increase was observed in insulin resistance and in serum insulin levels that relate to time since menopause rather than to the chronological age of patients [126,127]. After menopause, a close correlation between insulin resistance and the decreasing ovarian estrogen production has been consistently reported as risk factor for cardiovascular diseases and for malignancies [16,128].

Elevated fasting glucose (EFG) level is an easily accessible mirror reflecting the insulin resistance of patients. EFG was a strong predictor of breast cancer among estrogen deficient perimenopausal and postmenopausal cases but it was not similarly dangerous for young premenopausal women [20].In postmenopausal women, after age of 65 years, newly diagnosed breast cancer incidence showed strong positive association with their highly elevated blood glucose levels [129].

Central adiposity is associated to increased risk of breast, endometrial and colorectal cancers, particularly after menopause [110]. In obese postmenopausal women weight loss, regular physical activity or estrogen replacement alone has beneficial antidiabetogenic effect by improving the insulin sensitivity [93]. HRT use in women attenuates the obesity associated cancer risk, especially for the malignancies of breast and endometrium [130,131]. Recently, beneficial systemic changes; such as increased insulin sensitivity and elevated estrogen levels resulted in decreased oral cancer risk in women with moderate alcohol consumption [132].

In men the metabolic significance of estrogen environment has newly been recognized and today its role in male physiology seems also to be essential [8]. Sporadic male cases with complete estrogen deficiency exhibit severe type-2 diabetes being resistant to usual therapy but they may be treated by estrogen substitution. In powerlifters ingesting anabolic steroids the breakdown of sexual steroid balance may result in diminished glucose tolerance and insulin resistance [133]. Based on the findings found in women, a disturbed equilibrium of sexual steroids associated with insulin resistance may also be important cancer risk in men.

Conclusion

Thorough interplay between two systemic alterations; insulin resistance and estrogen deficiency may illuminate many apparently controversial experimental and clinical findings in oncology. Equilibrium of sexual steroid levels may be crucial for the health both in women and men. Correction of altered androgen to estrogen levels increases the insulin sensitivity, whereas treatment of insulin resistance may help to improve the sexual steroid equilibrium.

Interactions between insulin resistance and estrogen deficiency and their role in the initiation and progression of human malignancies may supply completely new strategies in primary cancer prevention and tumor therapy.

References

[1] Kahn CR, Folli F: Molecular determinant of insulin action. *Hormon Res.,* 39:93-101, 1993.

[2] Reaven GM: Banting lecture 1988: Role of insulin resistance in human disease. *Diabetes,*37:1595-1607, 1988.

[3] Suba Zs: Insulin resistance, hyperinsulinemia and cancer risk. Chapter 2, pp. 19-40. In: Estrogen versus Cancer. Nova Science Publishers Inc, New York, 2009.

[4] Björnström L, Sjöberg M: Mechanisms of estrogen receptor signaling: Convergence of genomic and nongenomic actions on target genes. *Mol. Endocrinol.,* 19:833-842, 2005.

[5] Reckelhoff JF: Sex steroids, cardiovascular disease, and hypertension. *Hypertension,* 45:170-174, 2005.

[6] Suba Zs: Insulin resistance, estrogen deficiency and cancer risk. Chapter 7. In: Estrogen versus Cancer. Nova Science Publishers Inc. New York, 2007.

[7] Ehrmann DA, Barnes RB, Rosenfield RL, Cavaghan MK, Imperial J: Prevalence of impaired glucose tolerance and diabetes in women with polycystic ovary syndrome. *Diabetes Care*, 22:141-146, 1999.

[8] Faustini-Fustini M, Rochira V, Carani C: Oestrogen deficiency in men: where are we today? *Eur. J. Endocrinol.*, 140:111-129, 1999.

[9] Schneider JG, Tompkins C, Blumenthal RS, Mora S: The metabolic syndrome in women. *Cardiol. Rev.,*14:286-291, 2006.

[10] Wu ShI, Chou P, Tsai ShT: The impact of years since menopause on the development of impaired glucose tolerance. *J. Clin. Epidemiol.*, 54:117-120, 2001.

[11] Nestler JE, Jakubowicz DJ, deVargas AF, Brik C, Quintero N, Medina F: Insulin stimulates testosterone biosynthesis by human thecal cells from women polycystic ovary syndrome by activating its own receptor and using inositolglycan mediators as the signal transduction system. *J. Clin. Endocrinol. Metab.*, 83:2001-2005, 1998.

[12] DeFronzo RA, Ferrannini E: Insulin resistance: a multifaceted syndrome responsible for NIDDM, obesity, hypertension, dyslipidemia and atherosclerotic cardiovascular disease. *Diabetes Care*, 14:173-194, 1991.

[13] Bloomgarden ZT: Second World Congress on the Insulin Resistance Syndrome: Mediators, pediatric insulin resistance, the polycystic ovary syndrome, and malignancy. *Diabetes Care*, 28:1821-1830, 2005.

[14] Wrighting Group for the Women's Health Initiative Investigators: Risks and benefits of estrogen plus progestin in healthy postmenopausal women: principal results from the Women's Health Initiative randomized controlled trial. *JAMA*,288:321-333, 2002.

[15] Suba Z: Gender-related hormonal risk factors for oral cancer. *Pathol. Oncol. Res.*, 13:195-202, 2007.

[16] Suba Z: Common soil of smoking-associated and hormone-related cancers: estrogen deficiency. *Oncol. Rev.,* 4:73-87, 2010.

[17] Ragaz J, Wilson K, Frohlich J, Muraca G, Budlovsky J: Dual estrogen effects on breast cancer: endogenous estrogen stimulates, exogenous estrogen protects. Further investigation of estrogen chemoprevention is warranted. *Cancer Res.*, 70(suppl 24):441, 2010.

[18] Gupta K, Krishnaswamy G, Karnad A, Peiris A: Insulin: A novel factor in carcinogenesis. *Am. J. Med. Sci.,* 323:140-145, 2002.

[19] Yu H, Rohan Th: Role of insulin-like growth factor family in cancer development and progression. *J. Natl. Cancer Inst.,* 92:1472-1489, 2000.

[20] Muti P, Quattrin T, Grant BJ, Krogh V, Micheli A, Schunemann HJ, Ram M, Freudenheim JL, Sieri S, Trevisan M, Berrino F: Fasting glucose is a risk factor for breast cancer. *Cancer Epidemiol. Biomark. and Prev.,* 11:1361-1368, 2002.

[21] Balkau B, Kahn H, HS: Hyperinsulinemia predicts fatal liver cancer but is inversely associated with fatal cancer at some other sites: The Paris Prospective Study. *Diabetes Care*, 24:843-849, 2001.

[22] McKeown-Eyssen: Epidemiology of colorectal cancer revisited: are serum triglycerides and/or plasma glucose associated with risk? *Cancer Epidemiol. Biomark. and Prev.*, 3:687-695, 1994.

[23] Yeung NG, Husain I, Waterfall N: Diabetes mellitus and bladder cancer. An epidemiological relationship? *Pathol. Oncol. Res.*, 9:30-31, 2003.

[24] Barnard RJ, Aronson WJ, Tymchuk CN, Ngo TH: Prostate cancer: another aspect of the insulin-resistance syndrome? *Obes. Rev.,* 3:303-308, 2002.

[25] Ujpál M, Matos O, Bibók Gy, Somogyi A, Szabó Gy, Suba Z: Diabetes and oral tumors in Hungary. Epidemiological correlations. *Diabetes care,* 27:770-774, 2004.

[26] Suba Z, Barabás J, Szabó Gy, Takács D, Ujpál M: Increased prevalence of diabetes and obesity in patients with salivary gland tumors. *Diabetes Care*, 28:228, 2005.

[27] Key TJ, Applyby PN, Reeves GK: Body mass index, serum sex hormones and breast cancer risk in postmenopausal women. *J. Natl. Cancer Inst.*, 95:1218-1226, 2003.

[28] Soliman PT, Oh JC, Schmeler KM, Sun CC, Slomovitz BM, Gershenson DM, Burke TW, Lu KH: Risk factors for young premenopausal women with endometrial cancer. *Obstet. Gynecol.,* 105:575-580, 2005.

[29] Cowey S, Hardy RW: The metabolic syndrome: A high-risk state for cancer? *Am. J. Pathol.*, 169:1505-1522, 2006.

[30] Beatson TG: On the treatment of inoperable cases of carcinoma of the mamma. Suggestion for a new treatment with illustrative cases. *Lancet,* 2:104-107, 1896.

[31] Berrino F, Muti P, Micheli A, Bolelli G, Krogh V, Scijano R et al.: Serum sex hormone levels after menopause and subsequent breast cancer. *J. Natl. Cancer Inst.,* 88:291-296, 1996.

[32] La Vecchia C, Brinton LA, McTiernan A: Menopause, hormone replacement therapy and cancer. *Maturitas,* 39:97-115, 2001.

[33] Feigelson HS, Henderson BE: Estrogens and breast cancer. *Carcinogenesis*, 17:2279-2284, 1996.

[34] Colditz GA, Hankinson SE, Hunter DJ, Willett, WC, Manson JE, Stampfer MJ et al: The use of estrogens and progestins and the risk of breast cancer in postmenopausal women. *N. Engl. J. Med.,* 332:1589-1593, 1995.

[35] Diamanti-Kandarakis E: Hormone replacement therapy and risk of malignancy. *Curr. Opinion Obstet. Gynecol.*, 16:73-78, 2004.

[36] Key TJ, Pike MC: The dose-effect relationship between 'unopposed' oestrogens and endometrial mitotic rate: its central role in explaining and predicting endometrial cancer risk. *Br. J. Cancer*, 57:205-212, 1988.

[37] Toniolo PG, Levitz M, Zeleniuch-Jacquotte A, Banerjee S, Koenig KL, Shore RE, Strax P, Pasternak BS: A prospective study of endogenous estrogens and breast cancer in post-menopausal women. *J. Natl. Cancer Inst.*, 86:1076-1082, 1995.

[38] Henderson, BE, Ross RK, Pike MC: Hormonal chemoprevention of cancer in women. *Science*, 259:633-638, 1993.

[39] Hulka BS, Liu ET, Lininger RA: Steroid hormones and risk of breast cancer. *Cancer*, 74:1111-1124, 1993.

[40] Pike M, Bernstein L, Spicer D: Exogenous hormones and breast cancer risk. In: Neiderhuber J (ed) Current Therapy in Oncol. BC Decker, St. Louis, MO, pp 292-302, 1993.

[41] Liehr JG: Is estradiol a genotoxic and mutagenic carcinogen? *Endocrine. Rev.*, 21:40-54, 2000.

[42] Greenwald P, Caputo TA, Wolfgang PE: Endometrial cancer after menopausal use of estrogens. *Obstet. Gynecol.,* 50:239-243, 1977.

[43] Rodriguez C, Patel AV, Calle EE, Jacob EJ: Estrogen replacement therapy and ovarian cancer mortality in a large prospective study of US women. *JAMA*, 285:1460-1465, 2001.

[44] Negri E, Tzonou A, Beral V et al: Hormonal therapy for menopause and ovarian cancer in a collaborative re-analysis of European studies. *Int. J. Cancer,* 80:848-851, 1999.

[45] Lacey JV, Mink PJ, Lubin JH, Sherman ME, Troisi R, Hartge P, Schatzkin A, Schairer C: Menopausal hormone replacement therapy and risk of ovarian cancer. *JAMA,* 288:334-341, 2002.

[46] International Agency for Research on Cancer: Monographs on the evaluation of carcinogenic risks to humans: hormonal contraception and postmenopausal hormone therapy. *IARC,* Lyon, France, vol. 72, 1999.

[47] Russo J, Fernandez SV, Russo PA, Fernbaugh R, Sheriff FS, Lareef HM, Garber J, Russo IH: 17-beta-estradiol induces transformation and tumorigenesis in human breast epithelial cells. *FASEB J.,* 20:1622-1634, 2006.

[48] Dickson RB, Gelmann EP, Knabbe C, Jasid K, Bates S, Swain S: Mechanisms of estrogenic and antiestrogenic regulation of growth of human breast carcinoma. In: Klijn JGM (ed): Hormonal manipulation of cancer: peptides, growth factors and new (anti)steroidal agents. Raven Press, New York, pp. 381-403, 1987.

[49] Katzenellenbogen BS: Estrogen receptors: bioactivity and interactions with cell signaling pathways. *Biol. Reprod.,* 54:287-293, 1996.

[50] Ames BN, Shigenaga MK, Gold LS: DNA lesions, inducible DNA repair and cell division: three key factors in mutagenesis and carcinogenesis. *Environ. Perspect.*, 101:35-44, 1993.

[51] Li JJ, Li SA: Estrogen carcinogenesis in hamster tissues: a critical review. *Endocr. Rev.,* 11:524-531, 1990.

[52] Nandi S: Role of hormones in mammary neoplasia. *Cancer Res.,* 38:4046-4049, 1978.

[53] Clark RB, Howell A, Potten CS, Anderson E: Dissociation between steroid receptor expression and cell proliferation in human breast. *Cancer Res.,* 57:4987-4991, 1997.

[54] Ashburn SP, Han X, Liehr JG: Microsomal hydroxylation of 2- and 4-fluorestradiol to catechol metabolites and their conversion to methyl ethers: Catechol estrogens as possible mediators of hormonal carcinogenesis. *Mol. Pharmacol.*, 43:534-541, 1993.

[55] Ursin G, London S, Stanczyk FZ, Gentzschein E, Paganini, Hill A, Ross RK, Pike MC: Ureinary 2-hydroxyestrone/16 alpha-hydroxyestrone ratio and risk of breast cancer in postmenopausal women. *J. Natl. Cancer Inst.*, 91:1067-1072, 1999.

[56] Salama SA, Kamel M, Awad M, Nasser AH, Al-Hendy A, Botting S, Arrastia C: Catecholestrogens induce oxidative stress and malignant transformation in human endometrial glandular cells: protective effect of Catechol-O-methyltransferase. *Int. J. Cancer*, 123:1246-1254, 2008.

[57] Tsutsui T, Barrett JC: Neoplastic transformation of cultured mammalian cells by estrogens and estrogen-like chemicals. *Environ. Health Perspect,* 105(suppl.3):619-624,1997.

[58] Banerjee SK, Banerjee S, Li SA, Li JJ: Induction of chromosome aberrations in Syrian hamster renal cortical cells by various estrogens. *Mutat. Res*., 311:191-197, 1994.

[59] Barrett JC, Wong A, McLachlan JA: Diethylstilbestrol induces neoplastic transformation without measurable gene mutation at two loci. *Science,* 212:1402-1404, 1981.

[60] Mobley JA, Bhat AS, Brueggemeier RW: Measurement of oxidative DNA damage by catechol estrogens and analogues in vitro. *Chem. Res. Toxicol.*, 12:270-277, 1999.

[61] Michos C, Kiortsis DN, Evangelou A, Karkabounas S: Antioxidant protection during menstrual cycle: the effects of estradiol on ascorbic-dehydroascorbic acid plasma levels and total antioxidant plasma status in eumenorrhoic women during menstrual cycle. *Acta Obstet. Gynecol. Scand.*, 85:960-965, 2006.

[62] Freedman ND, Lacey JV, Hollenbeck AR, Leitzmann MF, Schatzkin A, Abnet ChC: The association of menstrual and reproductive factors with upper gastrointestinal tract cancers in the NIH-AARP Cohort. *Cancer,* 116:1572-1581, 2010.

[63] McGrath M, Michaud DS, De Vivo I: Hormonal and reproductive factors and the risk of bladder cancer in women. *Am. J. Epidemiol.*, 163:236-244, 2006.

[64] La Vecchia C, D'Avanzo B, Franceschi S, Negri E, Parazzini F, Decarli A: Menstrual and reproductive factors and gastric-cancer in women. *Int. J. Cancer,* 59:761-764, 1994.

[65] Britt K, Ashworth A, Smalley M. Pregnancy and the risk of breast cancer. *Endocrine.-Related Cancer,* 14:907-933, 2007.

[66] Wolpert BJ, Amr S, Ezzat S, Saleh D, Gouda I, Loay I et al: Estrogen exposure and bladder cancer risk in Egyptian women. *Maturitas,* 67:353-357, 2010.

[67] Teras LR, Patel AV, Rodriguez C, Thun MJ, Calle EE: Parity, other reproductive factors, and risk of pancreatic cancer mortality in a large cohort of U.S. women. *Cancer Causes and Control*, 16:1035-40, 2005.

[68] Bosetti C, Negri E, Franceschi S, Conti E, Levi F, Tomei F, La Vecchia C: Risk factors for oral and pharyngeal cancer in women: a study from Italy and Switzerland. *Br. J. Cancer*, 82:204-207, 2000.

[69] Suba Zs: Estrogen deficiency as cancer risk factor. Chapter 5. pp: 85-106. In: Estrogen versus Cancer. Nova Science Publishers Inc, New York, 2009.

[70] Olsson H, Bladström AM, Ingvar C: Are smoking-associated cancers prevented or postponed in women using hormone replacement therapy? *Obstet. Gynecol.,* 102:565-570, 2003.

[71] Gallus S, Bosetti C, Franceschi S, Levi F, Simonato L, Negri E, La Vecchia C: Oesophageal cancer in women: tobacco, alcohol, nutritional and hormonal factors. *Br. J. Cancer,* 85:341-345, 2001.

[72] Parazzini F, La Vecchia C, Negri E, Franceschi S, Bolis G: Case-control study of estrogen replacement therapy and risk of cervical cancer. *Br. Med. J.,* 315:85-88, 1997.

[73] Fernandez E, Gallus S, Bosetti C, Franceschi S, Negri E, La Vecchia C: Hormone replacement therapy and cancer risk: a systematic analysis from a network of case-control studies. *Int. J. Cancer,* 105:408-412, 2003.

[74] Kreuzer M, Gerken M, Heinrich J, Kreienbrock L, Wichmann HE: Hormonal factors and risk of lung cancer among women? *Int. J. Epidemiol.*, 32:263-271, 2003.

[75] Anderson GL, Judd HL, Kaunitz AM, Barad DH, Beresford SA, Pettinger M, Liu J, McNeeley SG, Lopez AM: Women's Health Initiative Investigators. Effects of estrogen plus progestin on gynaecologic cancers and associated diagnostic procedures: The Women's Health Initiative randomized trial. *JAMA,* 290:1739-1748, 2003.

[76] Shapiro S: False alarm: postmenopausal hormone therapy and ovarian cancer. *Climacteric*, 10:466-470, 2007.

[77] Anderson GL, Limacher M, Assaf AR, Bassford T, Beresford SA, Black H, Bonds D et al. Women's Health Intitative Steering Committee. Effects of conjugated equine estrogen in postmenopausal women with hysterctomy: the Women's Health Intitative randomized controlled trial. *JAMA,* 291:1701-1712, 2004.

[78] LaCroix AZ, Chlebowski RT, Manson JE, Aragaki AK, Johnson KC, Martin L et al: Health outcomes after stopping conjugated equine estrogens among postmenopausal women with prior hysterectomy. A randomized controlled trial. *JAMA*, 305:1305-1314, 2011.

[79] Nilsson S, Makela S, Treuter E, Tujague J, Thomsen J, Andersson G, Enmark E, Pettersson K, Warner M, Gustafsson JA: Mechanisms of estrogen action. *Physiol. Rev.,* 81:1535-1565, 2001.

[80] Hall JM, McDonnell DP: The estrogen receptor β-isoform (ERβ) of the human estrogen receptor modulates ERα transcriptional activity and is a key regulator of the cellular response to estrogens and antiestrogens. *Endocrinol.,* 140:5566-5578, 1999.

[81] Segars J, Driggers P: Estrogen action and cytoplasmic signaling cascades. Part I: Membrane-associated signaling complexes. *Trends Endocrin. Metab.*, 13:349-354, 2002.

[82] Helguero LA, Faulds MH, Gustafsson JA, Haldosen LA: Estrogen receptors α (ERα) and β (ERβ) differentially regulate proliferation and apoptosis of the normal murine mammary epithelial cell line HC11. *Oncogene,* 24:6605-6616, 2005.

[83] Suba Zs: Antiestrogen or estrogen as anticancer drug. Ch. 4. In: Sex Hormones, Development, Regulation and Disorders. Hoffmann AB (ed). Nova Science Publishers Inc. New York, 2011.

[84] Razandi M, Pedram A, Greene GL, Levin ER: Cell membrane and nuclear estrogen receptors (ERs) originate from a single transcript: studies of ERα and ERβ expressed in Chinese hamster ovary cells. *Mol. Endocrinol.,* 13:307-319, 1999.

[85] Driggers PH, Segars JH: Estrogen action and cytoplasmic signaling pathways. Part II: The role of growth factors and phosphorylation in estrogen signaling. *Trends Endocrin. Metab.,* 13:422-427, 2002.

[86] Kato S, Endoh H, Masuhiro Y, Kitamoto T, Uchiyama S, Sasaki H, Masushige S, Gotoh Y, Nishida E, Kawashima H, Metzger D, Chambon P: Activation of the estrogen receptor though phosphorylation by mitogen-activated protein kinase. *Science,* 270: 1491-1494, 1995.

[87] Lundholt BK, Briand P, Lykkesfeldt AE: Growth inhibition and growth stimulation by estradiol of estrogen receptor transfected human breast epithelial cell lines involve different pathways.*Breast Cancer Res. Treat.,* 67:199-214, 2001.

[88] Massarweh S, Schiff R: Resistance to endocrine therapy in breast cancer: exploiting estrogen receptor/growth factor crosstalk. *Endocrin-Related Cancer Suppl.*, 13, 1:S15-24, 2006.

[89] Marquez-Garban DC, Chen HW, Fishbein MC, Goodglick L, Pietras RJ: Estrogen receptor signaling pathways in human non-small cell lung cancer. *Steroids*, 72:135-143, 2007.

[90] Nelson KG, Takahashi T, Bossert NL, Walmer DK, McLachlan JA: Epidermal growth factor replaces estrogen in the stimulation of female genital-tract growth and differentiation. Proceed. *Natl. Acad. Sci. USA* 88:21-25, 1991.

[91] Curtis SW, Washburn T, Sewall C, DiAugustine R, Lindzey J, Couse JF, Korach KS: Physiological coupling of growth factor and steroid receptor signaling pathway: estrogen receptor knockout mice lack estrogen-like response to epidermal growth factor. P*roceed. Natl. Acad. Sci. USA* 93: 12626-12630, 1996.

[92] Barros RPA, Machado UF, Gustafsson JA: Estrogen receptors: new players in diabetes mellitus. *Trends Molecular. Med.,* 9:425-431, 2006.

[93] Choi SB, Jang JS, Park S: Estrogen and exercise may enhance β-cell function and mass via insulin receptor substrate 2 induction in ovarectomized diabetic rats. *Endocrinology,* 146:4786-4794, 2005.

[94] Bryzgalova G, Gao H, Ahren B, Zierath JR, Galuska D, Steiler TL et al: Evidence that oestrogen receptor-alpha plays an important role in the regulation of glucose homeostasis in mice: insulin sensitivity in the liver. *Diabetologia,* 49:588-597, 2006.

[95] Welch RD, Gorski J: Regulation of glucose transporters by estradiol in the immature rat uterus. *Endocrinology,* 140:3602-3608, 1999.

[96] Godsland IF, Walton C, Stevenson JC: Impact of menopause on metabolism. In: Diamond MP, Naftolin K, Eds: Metabolism in the female life cycle. Pp. 171-189, Ares Seerono Symposia, Rome 1993.

[97] Jones ME,Thorburn AW, Britt KL, Hewitt KN, Wreford NG Proietto J, Oz OK, Leury BJ, Robertson KM, Yao S, Simpson ER: Aromatase-deficient (ArKO) mice have a phenotype of increased adiposity. *Proc. Natl. Acad. Sci. USA,* 97:12735-12740, 2000.

[98] Muraki K, Okuya S, Tanizawa Y: Estrogen receptor alpha regulates insulin sensitivity trough IRS-1 thyrosin phosphorylation in mature 3T3-L1 adipocytes. *Endocr. J.,* 53:841-851, 2006.

[99] Shi J, Simpkins JW: 17β-Estradiol modulation of glucose transporter 1 expression in blood-brain barrier. *Am. J. Physiol.,* 272:1016-1022, 1997.

[100] Rosenbaum D, Haber RS, Dunaif A: Insulin resistance in polycystic ovary syndrome: decreased expression of GLUT-4 glucose transporters in adipocytes. *Am. J. Physiol.,* 264:197-202, 1993.

[101] Nagira K, Sasaoka T, Wada T, Fukui K, Ikubo M, Hori S, Tsuneki H, Saito S, Kobayashi M: Altered subcellular distribution of estrogen receptor is implicated in

estradiol-induced dual regulation of insulin signaling in 3T3-L1 adipocytes. *Endocrinology,* 147:1020-1028, 2006.

[102] Leung KC, Johannson G, Leung GM, Ho KKY: Estrogen regulation of growth hormone action. *Endocrine. Rev.,* 25:693–721, 2004.

[103] Walsh BW, Schiff I, Rosner B, Greenberg L, Ravinkar V, Sacks FM: Effects of postmenopausal estrogen replacement on the concentrations and metabolism of plasma lipoproteins. *New England J. Med.,* 325:1196-1204, 1991.

[104] Hamden K, Carreau S, Ellouz F, Masmoudi H, El FA: Protective effect of 17beta-estradiol on oxidative stress and liver dysfunction in aged male rats. *J. Physiol. Biochem.,* 63:195-201, 2007.

[105] Croston GE, Milan LB, Marschke KB, Reichman M, Briggs MR: Androgen receptor-mediated antagonism of estrogen-dependent low density lipoprotein receptor transcription in cultured hepatocytes. *Endocrinology,* 138:3779-3786, 1997.

[106] Pallottini V, Bulzomi P, Galluzzo P, Martini C, Marino M: Estrogen regulation of adipose tissue functions: Involvement of estrogen receptor isoforms. *Infectious Disorders – Drug Targets,* 8:52-60, 2008.

[107] Macotela Y, Boucher J, Tran TT, Kahn CR: Sex and depot differences in adipocyte insulin sensitivity and glucose. *Diabetes,* 58:803-812, 2009.

[108] Poehlman ET, Toth MJ, Gardner AW: Changes in energy balance and body composition at menopause. *Ann. Intern. Med.,* 123:673-675, 1995.

[109] Suba Z: Correlations between obesity and risk for salivary gland tumors. *Cancer Res. J.,* 3:55-68, 2009.

[110] Calle EE, Kaaks R: Overweight, obesity and cancer: epidemiological evidence and proposed mechanisms. *Nat. Rev. Cancer,* 4:579-591, 2004.

[111] Baghaei F, Rosmond R, Westberg L, Hellstrand M, Eriksson E, Holm G, Björntorp P: The CYP19 gene and association with androgens and abdominal obesity in premenopausal women. *Obesity Res.,* 11:578-585, 2003.

[112] Björntorp P: The regulation of adipose tissue distribution in humans. *Int. J. Obes. Relat. Metab. Disord.,* 20:291-302, 1996.

[113] Sartor BM, Dickey RP: Polycystic ovarian syndrome and the metabolic syndrome. *Am. J. Med.,* 330:336-342, 2005.

[114] Cara JF, Rosenfield RL: Insulin-like growth factor I and insulin potentiate luteinizing hormone induced androgen synthesis by rat ovarian thecal-interstitial cells. *Endrocrinology,* 123:733-739, 1988.

[115] Attia GR, Rainey WE, Carr BR: Metformin directly inhibits androgen production in human thecal cells. *Fertil. Steril.,* 76:517-524, 2001.

[116] Moghetti P, Castello R, Negri C, Tosi F, Spiazzi GG, Brun E, Balducci R, Toscano V, Muggeo M: Insulin infusion amplifies 17-(alpha)-hydroxy- corticosteroid intermediates response to adrenocorticotropin in hyperandrogenic women: apparent relative impairment of 17,20-lyase activity. *J. Clin. Endocrinol. Metab.,* 81:881-886, 1996.

[117] Christakou C, Diamanti-Kandarakis E: Role of androgen excess on metabolic aberrations and cardiovascular risk in women with polycystic ovary syndrome. *Women's Health,* 4:583-594, 2008.

[118] Solomon CG, Hu FB, Dunaif A, Rich-Edwards J, Willett WC, Hunter DJ, Colditz GA, Speizer FE, Manson JE: Long or highly irregular menstrual cycles as a marker for risk of type-2 diabetes mellitus. *JAMA,* 286:2421-2426, 2001.

[119] Elting MW, Dorsen TJM, Bezemer PD, Schoemaker J: Prevalence of diabetes mellitus, hypertension and cardiac complaints in a follow-up study of a Dutch PCOS population. *Hum. Reprod.,* 16:556-560, 2001.

[120] Gadducci A, Gargini A, Palla E, Fanucchi A, Genazzani AR: Polycystic ovary syndrome and gynecological cancers: is there a link? *Gynecol. Endocrinol.*, 20:200-208, 2005.

[121] Pierpoint T, McKeigue PM, Isaacs AJ, Wild SH, Jacobs HS: Mortality of women with polycystic ovary syndrome at long-term follow-up. *J. Clin. Epidemiol.,* 51:581-586, 1998.

[122] King H, Rewers M: WHO Ad Hoc Diabetes Reporting Group: Global estimates for prevalence of diabetes mellitus and impaired glucose tolerance in adults. *Diabetes Care*, 21:157-177, 1993.

[123] Wilson PWE: Does estrogen reduce glycemic levels? *Diabetes Care,* 21:1585-1586, 1998.

[124] Hirose K, Toyama T, Iwata H, Takezaki T, Hamajima N, Tajima K: Insulin, insulin-like growth factor-1 and breast cancer risk in Japanese women. *Asian Pac. J. Cancer Prev.,* 4:239-246, 2003.

[125] Goodwin PJ, Boyd NF, Hanna W, Hartwick W, Murray D, Qizilbash A, Redwood S, Hood N, DelGiudice ME, Sidlofsky S, McGready D, Wilkinson R, Mahoney L, Connelly P, Page DL: Elevated levels of plasma triglycerides are associated with histologically defined premenopausal breast cancer risk. *Nutr. Cancer,* 27:284-292, 1997.

[126] Godsland IF: Oestrogens and insulin secretion. *Diabetologia*, 48:2213-2220, 2005.

[127] Proudler AJ, Felton CV, Stevenson JC: Aging and the response of plasma insulin, glucose and C-peptide concentrations to intravenous glucose in postmenopausal women. *Clin. Sci.,* 83:489-494, 1992.

[128] Gohlke-Barwolf C: Coronary artery disease: is menopause a risk factor? *Basic Res. Cardiol.,* 95:177-183, 2000.

[129] Rapp K, Schroeder J, Klenk J, Ulmer H, Concin H, Diem G, Oberaigner W, Weiland SK: Fasting blood glucose and cancer risk in a cohort of more than 140,000 adults in Austria. *Diabetologia,* 49: 945-952, 2006.

[130] Morimoto LM, White E, Chen Z, Chlebowski RT, Hays J, Lopez AM, Manson J, Margolis KL, Muti PC, Stefanick ML, McTiernan A: Obesity, body size and risk of postmenopausal breast cancer: the Women's Health Initiative (United States). *Cancer Causes Control*, 13:741-751, 2002.

[131] McCullough ML, Patel AV, Patel R, Rodriguez C, Feigelson HS, Bandera EV, Gansler T: Body mass and endometrial cancer risk by hormone replacement therapy and cancer subtype. *Cancer Epidemiol. Biomark. Prev.*, 17:73-79, 2008.

[132] Takács D, Koppány F, Mihályi S, Suba Z: Decreased oral cancer risk by moderate alcohol consumption in non-smoker postmenopausal women. *Oral Oncol.,* 47:537-540, 2011.

[133] Cohen JC, Hickman R. Insulin resistance and diminished glucose tolerance in powerlifters ingesting anabolic steroids. *J. Clin. Endocrinol Metab.,* 64:960-3, 1987.

In: Estrogen Prevention for Breast Cancer
Editor: Zsuzsanna Suba
ISBN: 978-1-62417-378-3

Chapter III

Dose Dependent Biphasic Effect of Alcohol on Estrogen Level and Cancer Risk

Zsuzsanna Suba
National Institute of Oncology, Department of Surgical and Molecular Pathology, Budapest, Hungary

Abstract

Alcohol has dose-dependent effects on insulin signaling, which may partially explain its biphasic impact on human health. Results of epidemiological studies suggest that mild to moderate alcohol intake is associated with advantageous metabolic effects, such as reduction of the prevalence of insulin resistance and its cardiovascular complications. Moderate alcohol intake is associated with the lowest risk of type-2 diabetes as compared with both abstinence and excessive drinking. Recent studies focused on the hormonal changes induced by moderate and excessive alcohol consumption but there are controversial associations between dose-related alcohol intake and cancer risk. Plenty of data suggested direct associations between estrogen levels and alcohol consumption in postmenopausal women. Considering the justified dose-related ambiguous effects of alcohol intake on insulin sensitivity, a similar biphasic alcohol effect on estrogen production may also be presumed. Case-control studies on cancers of the upper aerodigestive tract reported a U-shaped curve of alcohol dose-related cancer incidence, with lowest risk in light drinkers as compared with abstainers and heavy drinkers. Regular, moderate drinking in postmenopausal cases increases insulin sensitivity and serum estrogen levels as well. Gender-related prevalence of alcohol-associated oral tumors revealed that moderate alcohol intake caused stronger reduction in cancer incidence among postmenopausal women than among men. These results suggest an additional beneficial anticancer impact of restored estrogen level in estrogen deficient womenwho drink in moderation. Conversely,direct correlation between increased prevalence of breast cancers and either moderate or excessive regular alcohol intake was strongly suggested conferred by increased estrogen level in older women. Recently, results of animal experiments justified that estrogen administration does not mediate rather suppresses mammary carcinogenesis in alcohol consumers.

Introduction

Chronic alcohol consumption is considered as major risk factor for carcinogenesis. Alcohol-associated risk of cancer development depends decisively on the overall daily consumption and on the ethanol concentration of alcoholic beverages [1, 2].

Epidemiological data have identified regular alcohol intake as a significant risk factor for upper aerodigestive tract cancer, including cancers of the oral cavity, pharynx, larynx and esophagus [3, 4, 5, 6]. Increased cancer risk mediated by alcohol intake may be observed in case of gastric and colon cancer as well [4, 5]. By contrast, some studies justify that moderate alcohol intake is not a risk factor for gastrointestinal diseases, which are associated with excessive alcohol consumption [7].

Data on correlations between alcohol intake and tumors at other sites are fairly controversial. Cancer inducing mechanisms of alcohol on breast cancer are under debate, but elevated estrogen level is a presumed conferring factor [8]. Conversely, clinical studies did not support any association between moderate alcohol intake and the cancers of ovary, pancreas and lung [4,9,10].

In middle aged and elderly Swedish women, moderate alcohol consumption was associated with a decreased risk of renal cell carcinoma [11].

Exact mechanisms by which chronic alcohol ingestion initiates carcinogenesis are not known, nevertheless, animal experiments support the concept that ethanol in itself is not carcinogenic but under certain conditions may be a cocarcinogen or tumor promoter [12]. Concentrated drinks have chronic irritant impact on the oropharyngeal and gastrointestinal mucosa, which results in chronic inflammation, increased regenerative processes and the deliberation of cytokines.

Alcohol consumption may cause systemic alterations such as; increased lipid peroxidation, which serves as a marker of oxidative stress [13]. All these changes might be risks for malignancies at several sites [14].

Ethanol metabolism leads to the generation of acetaldehyde, which is carcinogenic and mutagenic factor, binds to DNA and proteins, destructs folates. Acetaldehyde can also be produced by oral and faecal bacteria. Smoking and poor oral hygiene may change oral bacterial flora and increase acetaldehyde formation [15]. Other mechanisms also considered for alcohol stimulated carcinogenesis include enhanced production of free radicals and activation of procarcinogens.

Recent studies focused on the biphasic, ambiguous metabolic and hormonal changes induced by moderate and excessive alcohol consumption [16, 17, 18, 19], which may partially illuminate the controversial associations between alcohol and cancer risk. Moreover, gender specific differences in alcohol associated morbidity and mortality seem also to be relevant in understanding correlations between ethanol intake and carcinogenesis [20, 21, 22, 23, 24, 25].

Ambiguous Biphasic Metabolic and Hormonal Effects of Moderate and Excessive Alcohol Consumption

Insulin resistance has close correlations with cancer risk. Alcohol has dose-dependent effects on insulin signaling, which may partially explain its biphasic impact on human health [17]. Prevalence of insulin resistance is low in moderate drinkers, whereas increased in excessive alcohol consumers [26].

Results of epidemiological studies suggest that mild to moderate alcohol intake is associated with advantageous metabolic effects, such as reduction of the prevalence of metabolic syndrome, type-2 diabetes mellitus (DM) and their cardiovascular complications [18]. Moderate alcohol intake (<20 g/die) improves lipid profile, increases insulin sensitivity and decreases both waist circumference and serum insulin level [26]. Circulatory HDL-cholesterol level shows parallel increase with moderate doses of alcohol intake, which may be associated with its cardioprotective effect. Serum triglyceride level does not increase in moderate drinkers, whereas an increased level can be found in excessive drinkers as compared with abstinent cases [27].

Moderate alcohol consumption has significant cardioprotective effect and reduced cardiovascular morbidity and mortality both in men and women [24]. Examination of correlations between alcohol consumption and all-cause mortality revealed that it was reduced by moderate alcohol intake in both genders; however this protective impact was stronger on women than on men [28].

In the past decade several large population studies have shown a U shaped relation between dose dependent alcohol consumption throughout adulthood and mortality for both men and women [24, 29, 30]. Moderate alcohol intake was associated with the lowest risk for insulin resistance and type-2 diabetes as compared with both abstinence and excessive drinking [18, 30, 31].

In middle aged male patients, the two extremes; namely complete abstinence and excessive alcohol intake are risks for insulin resistant states, whereas moderate drinking decreases the risk for insulin resistance showing a U-shaped relation [32]. In the elderly population, especially in women, lifetime alcohol consumption is associated with type-2 DM, cardiovascular diseases and other causes of mortality in a U-shaped fashion as well [24] Moderate alcohol consumption is associated with lower, whereas abstinence and excessive alcohol intake with a higher risk of morbidity and mortality in aged people.

Hormonal changes in postmenopausal women appear to be associated with an increased risk for the development of insulin resistance and its complications [33]. Among postmenopausal women serum glucose and insulin levels have been found to be higher than among premenopausal patients. Moreover, an increased prevalence of metabolic syndrome and type-2 DM has also been observed with ageing after menopause [33, 34].

Slight or moderate alcohol ingestion improves insulin sensitivity in postmenopausal women by elevated adiponectin levels and the improvement of lipid profile [16]. In women after menopause moderate alcohol consumption has a well-known cardioprotective effect, resulting from decreased coagulation activity, improvement of dyslipidemia and antioxidant capacity with decreased lipid oxidation [35]. In aged women the effect of alcohol intake on coronary heart disease, cancer incidence and cancer mortality was highly influenced by their smoking history [36]. Regular moderate alcohol consumption beneficially decreased both total and cardiovascular mortality among never smokers however; in current and former smokers an increased cancer incidence was registered. In older women with a constant body weight, moderate alcohol consumption reduces insulin resistance and bioavailable serum IGF-I level, which may advantageously lower the risk for cancer [37].

There are controversial data concerning possible associations between hormone levels and alcohol intake in postmenopausal women. Review of eight studies established that moderate alcohol consumption may increase blood estradiol levels in women after menopause. Regular, slight or moderate alcohol intake in postmenopausal cases advantageously increases the insulin sensitivity and endogenous serum estrogen levels as well [38,39,40]. These results suggested that elevated estrogen levels may confer the association between alcohol consumption and increased breast cancer risk. Nevertheless, some authors reason that associations between alcohol ingestion and the risk of breast cancer do not appear to be mediated by estrogens [8].

Deleterious interaction of insulin resistance and estrogen deficiency in non-drinking postmenopausal cases illuminates that metabolic syndrome and type-2 diabetes are higher cancer risk factors for them as compared with men [23, 25, 39, 41, 42].

Protective role of hormone replacement therapy (HRT) for smoking associated cancers, such as oral cancer, was justified among smoker postmenopausal women [43]. Beneficial anticancer effects of hormone treatment were reported against gastric, colorectal, cervical liver and lung cancers [44, 45, 46, 47] and there are many contradictions concerning the associations of HRT and hormone dependent cancers as well [48, 49]. Recent data showed that for well-selected women, HRT use is safe and protective against breast cancer risk and for many other diseases of aged women [50, 51, 52]. Considering the new aspects of postmenopausal hormone treatment, moderate alcohol intake may reduce cancer risk in postmenopausal women either by increased insulin sensitivity or through elevated estrogen levels [38, 39, 53].

Associations of Alcohol Consumption, Estrogen Level and Breast Cancer Risk

Results of epidemiological studies strongly suggest that both moderate and excessive regular alcohol intake exhibits consistent association with an increased prevalence of breast cancer [4, 54, 55]. On the other hand, alcohol consumption increases endogenous sexual steroid production in postmenopausal women [40]. These alcohol-associated changes were arbitrarily linked and elevated circulatory estrogen level was presumed to be the mediator of increased breast cancer risk in alcohol consumer women disregarding the dose-related differences.

Insulin and estrogen are in close interaction in the regulation of cell proliferation and carcinogenesis [56, 57]. Considering the justified dose-related ambiguous effects of alcohol intake on insulin sensitivity a similar biphasic alcohol effect on estrogen production may also be presumed. Thorough investigation of correlations between dose-related alcohol intake and circulatory estrogen level may reveal advantageous increase in hormone level in light-to-moderate drinkers, whereas decreased level in excessive drinker women.

Alcohol might increase estrogen levels through different pathways. In the liver, alcohol metabolism can lead to a decreased catabolism of sex steroids [58]. Another possible mechanism is that alcohol increases aromatase activity [59]. Increased production of androgen precursors by adrenal glands was also suggested as a pathway for increased estrogen synthesis [40].

Several studies investigated the effects of alcohol ingestion on endogenous sex steroid levels in postmenopausal women, however the results are conflicting. Self-reported alcohol consumption data reflect an increased risk of breast cancer [60], which suggests that these data are not reliable. Diversity of self-reported data suggests underreporting and does not reflect real values regarding cancer risk. By contrast, in randomized clinical trials known quantities of alcohol were administered and acute effects on hormone levels were measured [61, 62, 63].

Clinical trials most consistently showed that regular alcohol intake was associated with elevated estradiol level. Alcohol drinking and endogenous sex steroid levels have been related to breast cancer in a large meta-analysis study, which showed that with each 10 g/die alcohol consumption, the breast cancer risk of women increases by approximately 7% [60]. This finding supported the hypothesis that alcohol use may increase at least partially the risk of breast cancer via elevated endogenous sex steroid level. Unfortunately, there was no strict distinction and threshold value between moderate and excessive alcohol consumption data.

Effect of low-to-moderate alcohol intake on breast cancer incidence has been inconsistent despite the extensive investigation of associations between alcohol consumption and breast cancerrisk [19, 64, 65, 66]. Epidemiologic studies addressing the association of alcohol consumption with breast cancer consistently suggest a modest association and a dose-response relationship [67].

Low levels of alcohol consumption were associated with a small increase in breast cancerrisk, with the most consistent measure being cumulative alcohol intake throughout adult life [64, 65]. Conversely, some authors established that low-to-moderate alcohol intake is not associated with increased breast cancer risk [19, 66]. Slight-to-moderate alcohol consumption could not negatively affect the breast cancer specific mortality of women with invasive tumor; whereas, it decreased the risk of their mortality from other causes [68].

Considering the strong correlation between insulin resistance and breast cancer, beneficial increase in insulin sensitivity by moderate alcohol intake may not induce mammary carcinogenesis. Elevated fasting glucose level, metabolic syndrome and type-2 diabetes are high risk factors for malignant breast tumors [69,70] and these alterations are in close correlation with decreased hormonal level and/or a defective signal transduction pathway of estrogens [56, 57].

There are strong correlations between obesity and breast cancer risk as well [71]. Overweight and obesity are typical insulin resistant states and obesity associated breast cancer risk is fairly high in postmenopausal estrogen deficient cases never using HRT. Conversely, obesity in premenopausal women seems to be inversely associated with breast cancer incidence, suggesting a protective capacity of adiposity for breast cancer risk in young age. Controversial associations of obesity and breast cancer prevalence are discussed in Chapter 4.

Recent results of animal experiments justified that estrogen does not induces but rather suppresses mammary carcinogenesis. In ovariectomized obese mice, mammary tumor development deriving from T47-D human breast cancer cells was suppressed by estrogen supplementation but obesity without estrogen enhanced tumor growth [72]. In ovariectomized female mice alcohol consumption and obesity increased the growth of injected Met-1 mouse mammary cancer cells. By contrast, estrogen substitution enhanced insulin sensitivity, triggered the loss of body fat and suppressed tumor growth [73, 74].

These concordant experimental results suggest a counteraction between alcohol intake, obesity and estrogen effect on breast cancer development casting doubt on the misbelief that elevated estrogen level may confer the carcinogenic impact of alcohol consumption and obesity.

Alcohol Consumption, Hormonal Changes and Risk for Oral Cancer

Alcohol consumption is a strong cancer risk factor, especially for oral cavity and upper alimentary tract cancers [3,4,5]. The risk was thought to be strongly and directly related to the dose of alcohol intake [2,3,75].

Even moderate alcohol consumption was considered to cause significant increase in the cancer incidence of upper aerodigestive tract [76]. Some authors observed gender related differences as well, stronger associations between lifetime alcohol intake and the cancer risk of upper digestive tract among women than men [20, 21]. Further analysis identified that there is no threshold level of alcohol consumption below which no increased risk for cancer would be evident [5]. Conversely, an ambiguous biphasic impact of moderate and excessive alcohol intake on the risk of oral and oropharyngeal cancers has also been published [3, 77].

It has been shown, that insulin resistance and type-2 DM are high risk factors for malignant tumors at different sites [78]. Epidemiological studies conducted in Hungary and in India showed an increased prevalence of oral premalignant lesions among patients with type-2 diabetes [22, 79]. Oral cancer proved to be more frequent among insulin resistant patients with type-2 DM as compared with type-1 diabetes cases [79]. Associations between type-2 DM and risk of salivary gland tumors were also reported [80].

Literary data suggest that moderate alcohol intake may reduce the overall cancer risk in postmenopausal women either by increased insulin sensitivity or through increasing estrogen protection [23, 81].

Recent studies focus on the correlation between dietary effects and oral cancer risk. According to the results of Italian and Swiss publications, the so-called Mediterranean diet, which improves insulin resistance has beneficial anticancer effects and decreases the risk of oral cancer and other malignancies [82, 83]. Moderate drinking of red wine proved to be cancer protective even among heavy smokers, via its antioxidant and insulin sensitizing effects and resveratrol content [84, 85].

The aim of the present study was to clarify the dose-related risk of alcohol consumption for oral cancer by separated investigation on non-smoker male and female cases. Prevalence of elevated fasting glucose level associated with alcohol intake and its correlation with oral cancer risk was also studied.

Materials and Methods

Patients. 608 non-smoker inpatients (466 males and 142 females) with histologically confirmed squamous cell oral carcinomas at the Department of Oral and Maxillofacial Surgery of Semmelweis University Budapest were included into the study. The controls were non-smoker tumor-free adults (264 males and 142 females) who volunteered to participate in stomato-oncological screening in the same period of time. Data of oral cancer patients and their controls were collected by means of questionnaires and from case reports of the inpatients. All patients gave their informed consent to participate in the study.

Age of patients. Age of female patients was especially important in this study. For each female oral cancer case a tumor-free female control was chosen who matched the patient's age (within 6 months) at the time of cancer diagnosis. The mean age of control male patients was chosen so as to be within 1 year of the mean age of the male oral cancer cases.

Smoking habits. Patients and controls who claimed to have never smoked or to have quit smoking more than 10 years before were included into the examination as non-smokers.

Alcohol consumption. Examinations were focused on the alcohol consumption habits, regarding the type and alcohol volume of beverages, as well as the frequency of alcohol intake. Patients drinking only on special occasions were regarded as non-drinkers. Patients who claimed to consume alcoholic beverages containing presumably less than 25g alcohol/day (eg.: 1 bottle of beer, or 2dl of wine, or 0.5dl of spirit), 5-7 days/week were regarded as moderate drinkers. Patients claiming to consume alcohol regularly above the moderate level (25g/day) were regarded as excessive drinkers. Three fractions were recorded according to drinking habits: non-drinkers (ND), moderate drinkers (MD) and excessive drinkers (ED) in both the tumor bearing and control groups.

*Blood glucose levels.*Male and female cases among oral cancer patients and their controls were separately investigated. Based on blood glucose levels the patients were divided into three groups:

1. N: Normal blood glucose levels ($\leq$ 5.5 mmol/l).
2. EFG: Elevated fasting glucose levels (5.6-6.9 mmol/l).
3. DM: Diabetes mellitus ($\geq$ 7.0 mmol/l).

Patients in the second and third groups were regarded as insulin resistant (IR). Earlier diagnosed and treated DM cases were also included even in case of normal blood glucose level. No type-1 DM patient participated in the examinations.

In the newly diagnosed cases of glucose metabolism disorder fasting blood glucose levels were determined repeatedly within 4 days. All analytical measurements were made by means of Hitachi 717/912 automatic analyzers (Roche Diagnostics, Boehringer, Mannheim, Germany). The level was regarded as elevated only if it was repeatedly >5.5 mmol/l.

Menopausal history of female patients. Ratios of postmenopausal cases and the *mean* age at the onset of menopause in the oral cancer and age matched control groups were determined. Ratio and length of postmenopausal hormone replacement therapy were also registered.

Statistical methods. Associations of oral cancer incidence with various risk factors were obtained from conditional logistic regression analysis by means of odds ratios (OR) and their 95% confidence intervals (CI). The chi-square test was also used for comparative statistical analysis. Mean ages of different patient groups were compared by means of two-sided Student-t test. A probability level of 5% was taken as limit of statistical significance.

Results

Data of 608 newly diagnosed and histologically verified oral squamous cell carcinoma cases, 466 male and 142 female cases were analyzed. Mean age of female oral cancer patients upon admission was significantly higher as compared with male oral cancer cases (63,6 vs. 56,6) ($p<0,01$).

Alcohol Consumption

In the male oral cancer group nearly half of the cases were excessive alcohol consumers (41.8%), and moderate drinkers were in minority (7,1%) (Table 1). A significantly lower regular alcohol consumption rate was registered in the male control group (23.4%), ($p<0.05$) however, the great majority of these cases were excessive drinkers (18.0%) and the ratio of moderate drinkers was significantly lower (5.4%) ($p<0.05$) (Table 2). In men, excessive alcohol consumption proved to be a strong risk factor for oral cancer (OR:2.2), however moderate alcohol consumption elevated the cancer risk only moderately (OR:1.4).

In the female oral cancer group, the rate of regular alcohol consumption was significantly lower as compared with the male oral cancer group (15.4% vs. 48.9%; $p<0.01$). Among the female drinker oral cancer patients the excessive alcohol intake predominated (12.6%), whereas moderate alcohol consumption was low (2.8%) (Table 3). Regarding the female control cases, both the excessive and moderate alcohol consumption rates were low (2.1% vs. 4.2%) (Table 4). In women, excessive alcohol consumption proved to be a strong risk factor for oral cancer (OR:3.6), but moderate drinking lowered the tumor risk (OR:0.7).

Table l. Percentage of dose-related alcohol intake and elevated fasting glucose level among male OC patients

	Fasting glucose			Patients	
Alcohol intake	N	EFG	DM	ALL	IR
No	24.9 %	12.2%	13.9%	51.1%	26.2%
Moderate	2.8%	1.9%	2.4%	7.1%	4.3%
Excessive	22.3%	9%	10.5%	41.8%	19.5%
				100%	50%

Table 2. Percentage of dose-related alcohol intake and elevated fasting glucose level among male control patients

	Fasting glucose			Patients	
Alcohol intake	N	EFG	DM	ALL	IR
No	36.5%	19.3%	20.8%	76.6%	40.1%
Moderate	2%	1.1%	2.3%	5.4%	3.4%
Excessive	11.8%	2.3%	42%	18%	6.4%
				100%	49.9%

Table 3. Percentage of dose-related alcohol intake and elevated fasting glucose level among female OC patients

	Fasting glucose			Patients	
Alcohol intake	N	EFG	DM	ALL	IR
No	33%	24.6%	27.5%	85.3%	52.1%
Moderate	1.4%	0%	1.4%	2.8%	1.4%
Excessive	7.7%	2.1%	2.8%	12.6%	4.9%
				100%	58.4%

Table 4. Percentage of dose-related alcohol intake and elevated fasting glucose level among female control patients

	Fasting glucose			Patients	
Alcohol intake	N	EFG	DM	ALL	IR
No	56.3%	17.6%	19.7%	93.7%	37.3%
Moderate	1.4%	0.7%	2.1%	4.2%	2.8%
Excessive	0%	0.7%	1.4%	2.1%	2.1%
				100%	42.2%

Blood Glucose Levels

Groups with elevated blood glucose level (EFG and DM) were considered to be insulin resistant (IR), and were summarized for statistical analysis.

In the male oral cancer group the ratio of elevated glucose levels (IR) was quite similar to that of control men (50.0% vs. 49.9%) (Tables 1. and 2.). However, among female oral cancer cases the incidence of elevated blood glucose levels was significantly higher than among female controls (58.4% vs. 42.2%; p<0,01) (OR:1.6) thus elevated blood glucose levels proved to be an oral cancer risk factor among women (Tables 3. and 4.).

Menopausal History of Female Patients

Almost all female oral cancer patients were postmenopausal (96%), whereas nearly a quarter of the age matched tumor-free controls where premenopausal (24%) (p<0,05). Mean age at menopause was significantly lower among the female oral cancer patients (45.4 yrs) as compared with their tumor-free controls (51.3 yrs) (p<0,05). Postmenopausal hormone replacement therapy was very rare in both groups, 2 cases in the oral cancer group and 3 cases among the controls and its length was 1.5-2 years.

Discussion

In earlier Hungarian studies on pooled smoker and non-smoker cases a separate analysis on alcohol consumption, elevated fasting glucose and postmenopausal sex hormone deficiency in women proved to be strong risk factors affecting oral cancer incidence [23, 86]. On the other hand, moderate alcohol consumption showed certain correlation with oral cancer risk in men, but exhibited inverse association with risk among women [25]. These sex differences might be explained at least partly by the menopausal metabolic and hormonal changes in women with oral cancer [23, 87]. Moderate alcohol intake may reduce the risk of oral cancer in postmenopausal women either by increased insulin sensitivity or through elevated estrogen levels [25, 38, 39].

The present findings justify the beneficial systemic effects of moderate alcohol intake in non smoker cases in contrast to the classical view, according to which in women consumption of alcoholic beverages is one of the most important local risk factors for oral cancer, even in lower doses [20, 76].Alcohol consumption exhibited its dose-related biphasic effect on oral cancer risk. Light drinkers showed moderate oral cancer risk among men, whereas decreased oral cancer risk among women. Heavy drinkers exhibited high risk for oral cancer both in male and female cases. EFG proved to be a strong risk factor for oral cancer in predominantly postmenopausal women, whereas it did not affect the oral cancer risk in men.

Earlier case-control studies concerning cancers of the oral cavity exhibited a U-shaped curve, with lower risk in light drinkers as compared to abstainers [3, 77]. Similar results were published on the cancer of larynx in some categories of light drinkers, and on cancer of esophagus [3, 88, 89]. A lower risk for oral cancer was established in men who drank up to 1 drink per day as compared with abstinent cases [90]. Some studies have shown a higher risk of certain diseases in abstainers as compared with moderate drinkers [29, 91].

In conclusion, the findings of this study cast doubts on the hypothesis that women may be more vulnerable to alcohol induced carcinogenesis than men [20, 21]. Presumably, advantageous systemic effects of moderate alcohol intake may compensate the intraoral toxic impact of alcoholic beverages, especially in women. The beneficial systemic changes, namely the increased insulin sensitivity and elevated estrogen levels may explain the advantageous protective effects of light drinking in postmenopausal women [25]. These findings may also help to understand the U-shaped nature of alcohol-related cancer incidence in the upper aerodigestive tract that has been described by several authors [3, 77, 89, 91].

Conclusion

Literary data on correlations between alcohol intake and cancer risk at different sites show many controversies despite thorough investigations. Recent studies suggest that drinking associated cancer risk exhibits biphasic nature depending on the dose of alcohol consumption and its impact on insulin sensitivity.

In case of the tumors of upper aerodigestive tract strong correlation with alcohol intake was assumed to be associated with the local irritant and toxic effects of alcoholic beverages on mucosal surfaces. Conversely, in female breast, hormonal mechanisms mainly excessive estrogen production was presumed to be in strong correlation with alcohol induced carcinogenesis as local tissue irritation was excluded.

Discovery of insulin resistance as a base of human diseases yielded new possibilities for investigations of alcohol induced cancer initiation at the end of the past century. Alcohol induces a dose dependent biphasic effect on insulin sensitivity, which explains many correlations between the decreased prevalence of cardiovascular diseases, the lower rate of all-cause mortality and moderate drinking. Further conspicuous differences were observed in the alcohol associated morbidity and mortality of male and female cases suggesting a thorough interaction between ethanol and the metabolism of sexual steroids.

Insulin resistance proved to be an important initiator of carcinogenesis at several sites. This systemic risk factor exhibits proven associations with the initiation and progression of malignancies. Strong correlations among alcohol intake, insulin resistance and cancer risk were revealed concerning both so-called smoking associated and hormone-related tumors.

Moderate alcohol consumption increases insulin sensitivity, whereas excessive drinking provokes insulin resistance. These ambiguous effects of alcohol intake seem to be reflected in certain studies on the cancers of upper aerodigestive tract, namely a dose related U-shape relation between ethanol intake and cancer risk. Gender-related differences in the prevalence of alcohol-associated oral tumors revealed that moderate alcohol intake caused stronger reduction in cancer incidence among postmenopausal women than among men. These results suggest an additional beneficial anticancer impact of increased estrogen level in estrogen deficient women who are moderate drinkers.

Breast cancer risk is highly associated with metabolic and hormonal disorders. Cancers of the breast and colon were among the first tumors in case of which the high cancer risks of metabolic syndrome and type-2 diabetes were recognized. Effects of moderate and excessive alcohol intake on breast cancer incidence were blurred resulting in a concept of breast tumor risk directly increasing with enhanced alcohol doses and estrogen levels. Nevertheless, recent epidemiological and experimental results suggest that estrogen does not increase breast cancer risk, but is rather protective.

In conclusion, methodologically strong investigations will reveal that both smoking associated and hormone related cancers might show similar biphasic risks dependentupon moderate or excessive alcohol intake.

References

[1] Lubin JH, Purdue M, Kelsey K, Zhang ZF et al. Total exposure and exposure rate effects for alcohol and smoking and risk of head and neck cancer: a pooled analysis of case-control studies. *Am. J. Epidemiol.* 170:937-47, 2009.

[2] Altieri A, Bosetti C, Gallus S, Franceschi S, Dal Maso L, Talamini R, et al. Wine, beer and spirits and risk of oral and pharyngeal cancer: a case–control study from Italy and Switzerland. *Oral Oncology*40:904-909, 2004.

[3] Franceschi S, Talamini R, Barra S, Baron AE, Negri E, Bidoli E, et al. Smoking and drinking in relation to cancers of the oral cavity, pharynx, larynx and esophagus in northern Italy. *Cancer Res.*50:6502-7, 1990.

[4] Brown LM. Epidemiology of alcohol-associated cancers. *Alcohol* 35:161-68, 2005.

[5] Bagnardi V, Blangiardo M, La Vecchia C, Corrao G. Alcohol consumption and the risk of cancer: a meta-analysis. *Alcohol Researchand Health*25:263-70, 2001.

[6] Huang WY, Winn DM, Brown LM, Gridley G et al. Alcohol concentration and risk of oral cancer in Puerto Rico. *Am. J. Epidemiol.* 157:881-887, 2003.

[7] Taylor B, Rehm J, Gmel G. Moderate alcohol consumption and the gastrointestinal tract. *Dig. Dis.* 23:170-6, 2005.

[8] Longnecker MP, Tseng M. Alcohol, hormones and postmenopausal women. *Alcohol Health and Research World*22:185-89, 1998.

[9] Genkinger JM, Hunter DJ, Spiegelman D, Anderson KE et al. Alcohol intake and ovarian cancer risk: a pooled analysis of 10 cohort studies. *Br. J. Cancer* 94:757-62, 2006.
[10] Nishino Y, Wakai K, Kondo T, Seki N, Ito Y et al. Alcohol consumption and lung cancer mortality in Japanese men: results from Japan collaborative cohort (JACC) study. *J. Epidemiol.* 16:49-56, 2006.
[11] Rashidkhani B, Akesson A, Lindblad P, Wolk A. Alcohol consumption and risk of renal cell carcinoma: a prospective study of Swedish women. *Int. J. Cancer* 117:848-53, 2005.
[12] Poschl G, Seitz HK. Alcohol and cancer. *Alcohol and Alcoholism* 39:155-65, 2004.
[13] Hartman TJ, Baer DJ, Graham LB, Stone WL et al. Moderate alcohol consumption and levels of antioxidant vitamins and isoprostanes in postmenopausal women. *Eur. J. Clin. Nutr.* 59:161-168, 2005.
[14] Tsuji S, Kawai N, Tsuji M, Kawano S, Hori M. Review article: inflammation-related promotion of gastrointestinal carcinogenesis: a perigenetic pathway. *Aliment Pharmacol and Therapeutics*18:82-89, 2003.
[15] Kurkivuori J, Salaspuro V, Kaihovaara P et al. Acetaldehyde production from ethanol by oral streptococci. *Oral Oncol.* 43:181-186, 2007.
[16] Joosten MM, Beulens JWJ, Kersten S et al. Moderate alcohol consumption increases insulin sensitivity and ADIPOQ expression in postmenopausal women: a randomized, crossover trial. *Diabetologia*51:1375-81, 2008.
[17] He L, Marecki JC, Serrero G, Simmen FA et al. Dose-dependent effects of alcohol on insulin signaling: Partial explanation for biphasic alcohol impact on human health. *Mol. Endocrinol.* 21:2541-2550, 2007.
[18] Beulens JW, Stolk RP, van der Schouw YT et al. Alcohol consumption and risk of type 2diabetes among older women. *Diabetes Care* 28:2933-8, 2005.
[19] Pellucchi C, Tramacere I, Boffetta P, Negri E, La Vecchia C. Alcohol consumption and cancer risk. *Nutr. Cancer* 63:983-990, 2011.
[20] Maier H, Tisch M, Conradt C, Pötschke- Langer M: Alcohol drinking and cancer of the upper aerodigestive tract in women. *Dtsch. Med. Wochenschr.* 124:851-4, 1999.
[21] Weikert C, Dietrich T, Boeing H, Bergmann MM, Boutron-Ruault MC, Clavel-Chapelon F et al.: Lifetime and baseline alcohol intake and risk of cancer of the upper aero-digestive tract in the European Prospective Investigation into Cancer and Nutrition (EPIC) study. *Int. J. Cancer* 125:406-12, 2009.
[22] Dikshit RP, Ramadas K, Hashibe M, Thomas G, Somanathan T, Sankaranarayanan R. Association between diabetes mellitus and pre-malignant oral diseases: a cross sectional study in Kerala, India. *Internat.J. Cancer* 118:453-57, 2006.
[23] Suba Z. Gender-related hormonal risk factors for oral cancer. *Pathol. Oncol. Res.* 13:195-202, 2007.
[24] Murray RP, Connett JE, Tyas SL, Bond R, Ekuma O, Silversides CK, et al. Alcohol Volume, Drinking Pattern, and Cardiovascular Disease Morbidity and Mortality: is there a U-shaped function? *Am. J. Epidemiol.* 155:242-47, 2002.
[25] Takács D, Koppány F, Mihályi S, Suba Z: Decreased oral cancer risk by moderate alcohol consumption in non-smoker postmenopausal women. *Oral Oncol.* 47:537-540, 2011.

[26] Freiberg MS, Cabral HJ, Heeren TC, Vasan RS, Ellison RC. Alcohol consumption and the prevalence of the metabolic syndrome in the U.S. A cross-sectional analysis of data from the Third National Health and Nutrition Examination Survey. *Diabetes Care* 27:2954-59, 2004.

[27] Pownall HJ, Ballantyne ChM, Kimball KT et al. Effect of moderate alcohol consumption on hypertriglyceridemia. *Arch. Intern. Med.* 159:981-987, 1999.

[28] Rostron B. Alcohol consumption and mortality risks in the USA. *Alcohol* Jan 25 [Epub ahead of print] 2012.

[29] Marmot MG, Rose G, Shipley MJ, Thomas BJ. Alcohol and mortality: a U-shaped curve. *Lancet* 1(8230):580-83, 1981.

[30] Grønbaek M, Deis A, Sorensen T, Becker U, Schnohr P, Jensen G. Mortality associated with moderate intakes of wine, beer, or spirits. *BMJ* 310:1165-69, 1995.

[31] Hendriks HF. Moderate alcohol consumption and insulin sensitivity: observations and possible mechanisms. *Annals Epidemiol.* 17:40-42, 2007.

[32] Sierksma A, Patel H, Ouchi N, Kihara S, Funahashi T, Heine RJ, et al. Effect of moderate alcohol consumption on adiponectin, tumor necrosis factor alpha and insulin sensitivity. *Diabetes Care* 27:184-89, 2004.

[33] Schneider JG, Tompkins C, Blumenthal RS, Mora S. The metabolic syndrome in women. *Cardiology in Review* 14:286-91, 2006.

[34] Wu SI, Chou P, Tsai ST. The impact of years since menopause on the development of impaired glucose tolerance. *J. Clin. Epidemiol.* 54:117-20, 2001.

[35] Rimm EB, Williams P, Fosher K, Criqui M, Stampfer MJ. Moderate alcohol intake and lower risk of coronary heart disease: meta-analysis of effects on lipids and hemostatic factors. . *BMJ* 319:1523-28, 1999.

[36] Ebbert JO, Janney CA, Sellers TA et al. The association of alcohol consumption with coronary heart disease mortality and cancer incidence varies by smoking history. *J. General. Intern. Med.* 20:14-20, 2005.

[37] Lavigne JA, Baer DJ, Wimbrow HH, Albert PS, Brown ED, Judd JT, et al. Effects of alcohol on insulin-like growth factor I and insulin-like growth factor binding protein 3 in postmenopausal women. *Am. J. Clin. Nutr.* 81:503-07, 2005.

[38] McDivit AM, Greendale GA, Stanczyk FZ, Huang MH. Effects of alcohol and cigarette smoking on change in serum estrone levels in postmenopausal women randomly assigned to fixed doses of conjugated equine estrogens with or without a progestin. *Menopause* 15:382-85, 2008.

[39] Purohit V. Moderate alcohol consumption and estrogen levels in postmenopausal women: a review. *Alcoholism: Clin. Exp. Res.* 22:994-97, 1998.

[40] Onland-Moret NC, Peeters PH, van der Schouw YT et al. Alcohol and endogenous sex steroid levels in postmenopausal women: a cross-sectional study. *Clin. Endocrinol. Metab.* 90:1414-19, 2005.

[41] Eliasson B, Attval S, Taskinen MR, Smith U. The insulin resistance syndrome in smokers is related to smoking habits. *Arterioscler. Thromb.* 14:1946-50, 1994.

[42] Augustin L, Gallus S, Negri E, La Vecchia C. Glycemic index, glycemic load and risk of gastric cancer. *Annals Oncol.* 15:581-584, 2004.

[43] Olsson H, BladströmAM, Ingvar C. Are smoking-associated cancers prevented or postponed in women using hormone replacement therapy? *Obstet. Gynecol.* 102:565-70, 2003.

[44] Camargo MC, Goto Y, Zabaleta J et al. Sex hormones, hormonal interventions and gastric cancer risk: a meta-analysis. *Cancer Epidemiol. Biomarkers Prev.*Oct 25 [Epub ahead of print] 2011.

[45] Fernandez E, Gallus S, Bosetti C, Franceschi S, Negri E, La Vecchia C. Hormone replacement therapy and cancer risk: a systematic analysis from a network of case-control studies. *Internat. J .Cancer* 105:408-12, 2003.

[46] La Vecchia C, D'Avanzo B, Franceschi S, Negri E, Parazzini F, Decarli A. Menstrual and reproductive factors and gastric-cancer risk in women. *Internat. J. Cancer* 59:761-64, 1994.

[47] Parazzini F, La Vecchia C, Negri E, Franceschi S, Moroni S, Chatenoud L, et al. Case-control study of estrogen replacement therapy and risk of cervical cancer. *BMJ* 315:85-88, 1997.

[48] Ettinger B, Friedman GD, Bush T, Quesenberry CPJ. Reduced mortality associated with long-term postmenopausal estrogen therapy. *Obstetrics Gynecol.*87:6-12, 1996.

[49] Grodstein F, Clarkson TB, Manson JE. Understanding the divergent data on postmenopausal hormone therapy. *New Engl. J. Med.* 348:645-50, 2003.

[50] Anderson GL, Limacher M, Assaf AR, Bassford T, Beresford SA, Black H, Bonds D et al. Women's Health Intitative Steering Committee. Effects of conjugated equine estrogen in postmenopausal women with hysterctomy: the Women's Health Intitative randomized controlled trial. *JAMA* 291:1701-1712, 2004.

[51] Ragaz J, Wilson K, Frohlich J, Muraca G, Budlovsky J: Dual estrogen effects on breast cancer: endogenous estrogen stimulates, exogenous estrogen protects. Further investigation of estrogen chemoprevention is warranted. *Cancer Res.*70:(24 suppl) 441, 2010.

[52] LaCroix AZ, Chlebowski RT, Manson JE, Aragaki AK, Johnson KC, Martin L et al: Health outcomes after stopping conjugated equine estrogens among postmenopausal women with prior hysterectomy. A randomized controlled trial. *JAMA* 305:1305-1314, 2011.

[53] Suba Z: Common soil of smoking-associated and hormone-related cancers: estrogen deficiency. *Oncol. Rev.* 4:73-87, 2010.

[54] Terry MB, Zhang FF, Kabat G, Britton JA et al. Lifetime alcohol intake and breast cancer risk. *Ann. Epidemiol.* 16:230-240, 2006.

[55] Stolzenberg-Solomon RZ, Chang SC, Leitzmann MF et al. Folate intake, alcohol use and postmenopausal breast cancer risk in the Prostate, Lung, Colorectal and ovarian Cancer Screening Trial. *Am. J. Clin. Nutr.* 83:895-904, 2006.

[56] Suba Z. Interplay between insulin resistance and estrogen deficiency as co-activators in carcinogenesis. *Pathol. Oncol. Res.* 18:123-133, 2012

[57] Suba Z, Kásler M. Interactions of insulin and estrogen in the regulation of cell proliferation and carcinogenesis. *Orv. Hetil.* 153:125-136, 2012.

[58] Sarcola T, Adlercreutz H, Heinonen S et al. The role of the liver in the acute effect of alcohol on androgens in women. *J. Clin. Endocrinol. Metab.* 86:1981-1985, 2001.

[59] Gavaler JS, Van Thiel DH. The association between moderate alcoholic beverage consumption and serum estradiol and testosterone levels in normal postmenopausal women: relationship to the literature. *Alcohol. Clin. Exp. Res.* 16:87-92, 1992.

[60] Hamajima N, Hirose K, Tajima K, Rohan T et al. Alcohol, tobacco and breast cancer – collaborative reanalysis of individual data from 53 epidemiological studies, including 58 515 women with breast cancer and 95 067 women without the disease. *Br. J. Cancer* 87:1234-45, 2002.

[61] Dorgan JF, Baer DJ, Albert PS, Judd JT et al. Serum hormones and the alcohol-breast cancer association in postmenopausal women. *J. Natl. Cancer Inst.* 93:710-715, 2001.

[62] Ginsburg ES, Walsh BW, Gao X, Gleason RE et al. The effect of acute ethanol ingestion on estrogen levels in postmenopausal women using transdermal estradiol. *J. Soc. Gynecol. Invest.* 2:26-29, 1995.

[63] Ginsburg ES, Mello NK, Mendelson JH, Barbieri RL et al. Effects of alcohol ingestion on estrogens in postmenopausal women. *JAMA* 276:1747-1751, 1996.

[64] Chen WY, Rosner B, Hankinson SE et al. Moderate alcohol consumption during adult life, drinking patterns and breast cancer risk. *JAMA* 306:1884-90, 2011.

[65] Mørch LS, Johansen D, Thygesen LC, Tjønneland A, Løkkegaard E, Stahlberg C, Grønbaek M. Alcohol drinking, consumption patterns and breast cancer among Danish nurses: a cohort study. *Eur. J. Public Health* 17:624-9, 2007.

[66] Zhang M, Holman CD. Low-to-moderate alcohol intake and breast cancer risk in Chinese women. *Br. J. Cancer* 105:1089-95, 2011.

[67] Coronado GD, Beasley J, Livaudais J. Alcohol consumption and risk of breast cancer. *SaludPublicaMex* 53:4407, 2011.

[68] Harris HR, Berquist L, Wolk A. Alcohol intake and mortality among women with invasive breast cancer. *Br. J. Cancer* 106:592-595, 2012.

[69] Muti P, Quattrin T, Grant BJ, Krogh V, Micheli A, Schunemann HJ, Ram M, Freudenheim JL, Sieri S, Trevisan M, Berrino F: Fasting glucose is a risk factor for breast cancer. *Cancer Epidemiol. Biomark. Prev.* 11:1361-1368, 2002.

[70] Bloomgarden ZT: Second World Congress on the Insulin Resistance Syndrome: Mediators, pediatric insulin resistance, the polycystic ovary syndrome, and malignancy. *Diabetes Care* 28:1821-1830, 2005.

[71] Rose DP, Vona-Davis L: Interaction between menopausal status and obesity in affecting breast cancer risk. *Maturitas*66:33-38, 2010.

[72] Nkhata KJ, Ray A, Dogan S Grande JP et al. Mammary tumor development from T47-D human breast cancer cells in obese ovariectomized mice with and without estradiol supplements. *Breast Cancer Res. Treat.* 114:71-83, 2009.

[73] Hong J, Holcomb VB, Kushiro, Núnez NP. Estrogen inhibits the effect of obesity and alcohol on mammary tumors and fatty liver. *Int. J.Oncol.* 39:1443-53, 2011.

[74] Holcomb VB, Hong J, Núnez NP. Exogenous estrogen protects mice from the consequences of obesity and alcohol. *Menopause* Jan 6 [Epub ahead of print] 2012.

[75] Fioretti F, Bosetti C, Tavani A, Franceschi S, La Vecchia C. Risk factors for oral and pharyngeal cancer in never smokers. *Oral Oncol.* 35:375-78, 1999.

[76] Barra S, Franceschi S, Negri E, Talamini R, La Vecchia C. Type of alcoholic beverage and cancer of the oral cavity, pharynx and oesophagus in an Italian area with high wine consumption. *Int. J. Cancer* 46:1017-20, 1990.

[77] Merletti F, Boffetta P, Ciccone G, Mashberg A, Terracini B. Role of tobacco and alcoholic beverages in the etiology of cancer of the oral cavity/oropharynx in Torino, Italy. *Cancer Res.* 49:4919-24, 1989.

[78] Verlato G, Zoppini G, Bonora E, Muggeo M. Mortality from site-specific malignancies in type 2 diabetic patients from Verona. *Diabetes Care* 26:1047-51, 2003.

[79] Ujpál M, Matos O, Bíbok G, Somogyi A, Szabó G, Suba Z. Diabetes and oral tumors in Hungary: Epidemiological correlations. *Diabetes Care* 27:770-74, 2004.

[80] Suba Z, Barabás J, Szabó G, Takács D, Ujpál M. Increased prevalence of diabetes and obesity in patients with salivary gland tumors. *Diabetes Care.* 28:228, 2005.

[81] SubaZs. Insulin resistance, hyperinsulinemia and cancer risk. Chapter 2. In: *Estrogen versus Cancer*. Nova Science Publishers, Inc. New York, 2009.

[82] Franceschi S, Favero A, Conti E, Talamini R, Volpe R, Negri E, et al. Food groups, oils and butter, and cancer of the oral cavity and pharynx. *Br. J. Cancer* 80:614-20, 1999.

[83] Kreimer AR, Randi G, Herrero R, Castellsague X, La Vecchia C, Franceschi S. Diet and body mass, and oral and oropharyngeal squamous cell carcinomas: Analysis from the IARC multinational case control study. *Int. J. Cancer* 118:2293-97, 2006.

[84] Bianchini F, Vainio H. Wine and resveratrol: mechanisms of cancer prevention? Review. *Eur. J. Cancer Prev.* 12:417-425, 2003.

[85] Petti S, Scully C. Association between different alcoholic beverages and leukoplakia among non- to moderate-drinking adults: a matched case-control study. *Eur. J. Cancer* 42:521-527, 2006.

[86] SubaZs. Insulin resistance and oral cancer risk. Chapter 4. pp. 77-97. In: *Horizons in Cancer Research.* Vol 43. ed: Watanabe HS. Nova Science Publishers Inc. New York. 2011.

[87] SubaZs. Systemic risk factors for oral cancer: Estrogen deficiency and insulin resistance. Chapter 7. pp. 143-156. In: *Progress in oral cancer research.* Ed: Nielsen FL. Nova Science Publishers Inc. New York 2008.

[88] De Stefani E, Mugnoz N, Estéve J, Vasallo A, Victora CG, Teuchmann S. Maté drinking, alcohol, tobacco, diet, and esophageal cancer in Uruguay. *Cancer Res.* 50:426-31, 1990.

[89] Falk RT, Pickle LW, Morris BL, Brown LM, Mason TJ, Buffler PA, Fraumeni JF Jr. Effect of smoking and alcohol consumption on laryngeal cancer risk in coastal Texas. *Cancer Res.* 49:4024-2, 1989.

[90] Boffetta P, Garfinkel L. Alcohol drinking and mortality among men enrolled in an American Cancer Society prospective study. *Epidemiol.*1:342-48, 1990.

[91] Kjaerheim K, Andersen A, Helseth A. Alcohol abstainers: a low-risk group for cancer - a cohort study of Norwegian teetotalers. *Cancer Epidemiol.Biomark. Prev. 2*:93-97, 1993.

In: Estrogen Prevention for Breast Cancer
Editor: Zsuzsanna Suba
ISBN: 978-1-62417-378-3

Chapter IV

Estrogen Level May Be Protective for Breast Cancer in Obese Women

Zsuzsanna Suba
National Institute of Oncology, Department of Surgical and Molecular Pathology. Budapest, Hungary

Abstract

Literary data suggest apparently ambiguous interaction between menopausal status and obesity-associated breast cancer risk. Before menopause, adiposity seem to exhibit a protective effect supposedly by defective estrogen-synthesis. By contrast, in postmenopausal cases obesity means a strong risk factor for breast cancer presumably conferred by an excessive estrogen-production of their adipose-tissue mass. Obesity and breast cancer risk are not in direct correlation; rather adiposity-associated metabolic and hormonal alterations may mediate inclination to malignancies. Neither body mass index nor abdominal circumference measurements could define the severity of insulin-resistance and defective estrogen-synthesis so their values in prophesying the risk of breast cancer are not reliable. Obesity is a pathologic state and endangers the healthy equilibrium of sexual hormone-production and regular menstrual cycles, which are prerequisites not only for reproduction, but also for somatic health in women.

In the majority of premenopausal women, obesity associated insulin-resistance may be counteracted by their preserved circulatory estrogen-level, consequently, not obesity but rather sufficient estrogen-level may be breast cancer protective. In obese old women, never using hormone replacement therapy (HRT) the breast cancer risk is high, which is associated to their deepening estrogen loss and increasing insulin-resistance.

By contrast, in fat postmenopausal women using HRT the risk of breast cancer is decreased. The protective effect of estrogen-substitution may counteract to obesity-associated insulin-resistance, similarly like in the majority of obese young women; the preserved circulatory levels of estrogen are beneficial. Correlations between continuous decrease in serum estrogen-level and increasing breast cancer risk during women's life should advance understanding breast cancer etiology and promote primary prevention measures.

Introduction

Many studies support apparently Janus-faced ambiguous interaction between menopausal status and obesity-associated breast cancer risk [1,2,3]. In young women, before menopause the level of adiposity seem to exhibit an inverse relation to breast cancer risk suggesting a protective effect of excessive fatty tissue deposition [1,4,5]. By contrast, in postmenopausal cases, particularly in the elderly, the association is highly positive, obesity seems to confer a strong risk for breast cancer [2,6]. Literary data suggest a quite inverse behavior of excessive adipose tissue in obese women, depending on their menopausal status. Controversial results of clinical studies suggest that obesity is associated with defective estrogen synthesis in young [7] and excessive estrogen production in older women [8,9].

Explanations for this presumed ambiguous correlation are based on the concept that high estrogen levels, either endogenous or exogenous, play crucial role in mammary carcinogenesis [10]. Supposedly, in obese postmenopausal women, high breast cancer risk may be conferred by the excessive estrogen production of their voluminous adipose tissue with consequently elevated circulating bio-available hormone level [11]. Nevertheless, several authors could find confusing and disturbing associations between obesity and breast cancer risk in women after menopause. Obese postmenopausal women, who had never used hormone replacement therapy (HRT) exhibited fairly high breast cancer risk [12]. By contrast HRT use attenuates or abolishes their increased cancer incidence [13,14,15] suggesting a protective impact of female sexual hormones in aged obese women.

In premenopausal cases, the presumed protective effect of obesity for breast cancer is less well understood and many authors attempt to clarify its mechanism. Results of clinical studies justify that in hormonally active young women, obesity induces mild or moderate decrease in circulating estrogen levels depending on the severity of insulin resistance [7]. Defective estrogen synthesis of obese premenopausal women may be reflected by their inclination to anovulatory infertility and long or irregular menstrual cycles [16]. Based on the concept of estrogen induced mammary carcinogenesis, obesity associated estrogen deficiency seem to justify the breast cancer preventive impact in fat premenopausal women.

Considering the whole spectrum of unexplained, apparently ambiguous biological behavior between breast cancers arising in premenopausal and postmenopausal women the existence of two distinct types of breast malignancieswas presumed occurring before and after menopause [17,18].

Obesity is a well-known cancer risk factor associated with different grades of insulin resistance and disturbance of male to female circulatory sexual steroid levels [19,20]. Hyperinsulinemia, dyslipidemia, elevated fasting glucose level and type-2 diabetes are the well documented concomitants of adiposity associated insulin resistance [21,22]. Obesity provokes further alterations in the endocrine system as well, conferred by an excessive circulatory androgen level at the expense of defective estrogen synthesis [23]. Nevertheless, the health benefit of pathologic states; such as overweight and obesity can hardly be justified at any age of women.

Even greatest studies, which equivocally strengthen the protective effect of obesity for premenopausal breast cancer risk, confess that the responsible mechanisms are completely obscure. Evidences from clinical endocrinological studies regarding correlations between defective hormonal status of obese women and decreased breast cancer incidence are inconsistent or fairly contradictory [1].

The aim of the present study is to clarify the realistic correlations between breast cancer risk and obesity-associated metabolic and hormonal alterations during the whole life of women. These associations are examined in an analytical reviewbased on the results of prospective, case-control and meta-analytic studies.

Grade and Distribution of Fat Deposition and Breast Cancer Risk

Diversity of methods concerning the measurement of obesity grade is confounding. Most important data characterizing the obesity grade are body mass index (BMI) [4,5,24] weight in kg [25,26,27] and circumference measurements; such as hip (HC), waist (WC) and waist to hip ratio (WHR) [14,28,29,30,31,32,33,34]. BMI and weight in kilogram reflects general adiposity, whereas the circumferences of waist and hip as well as their ratio should inform about the regional distribution of fatty tissue deposition. These circumference measurements aim to characterize the mass of visceral abdominal fat reflecting the grade of insulin resistance [34].

Fat deposition is thoroughly affected by male to female sexual steroid level [35]. In men, visceral adiposity with high abdominal circumference is typical. In obese premenopausal women, there are diverse possibilities for body fat distribution depending on their hormonal and metabolic status. Healthy estrogen predominance is associated with gluteofemoral fat deposition. These women may have slender waist, high HC and low WHC ratio. By contrast, in insulin resistance, hyperinsulinemia and excessive circulating male sexual steroids will produce abdominal adiposity in obese young women. Visceral fat deposition in women exhibits high WC lower HC with high WHC ratio. After menopause with decreasing estrogen level every year confers higher risk for insulin resistance [36,37]. Postmenopausal obesity is typically associated with visceral adiposity, especially in cases never using HRT.

Knowing the hormonal and metabolic background of the diverse types of obesity, BMI or body weight in kilogram may not correctly reflect the correlations among adiposity, insulin resistance and breast cancer risk in young women [14]. Nevertheless, till now, there are many studies trying to strengthen the protective effect of BMI defined obesity for breast cancer risk in premenopausal cases [2,4,5]. By contrast, low BMI among very young women could not significantly affect the premenopausal breast cancer risk in further studies [18].

Clinical results reflect fairly controversial associations between breast cancer risk and circumference-related obesity measurements as well. Some authors reported on the value of WC, HC and WHC ratio in prediction of premenopausal breast cancer occurrence [28,33]. Out of these data high WHC ratio seemed to be the most informative measurement as it presumably reflects the extent of intra-abdominal adiposity and the associated insulin resistance [33]. Further studies found exclusively the HC or WC value as relevant anthropometric predictors for breast cancer risk [14,28]. Surprisingly, high HC was directly associated with premenopausal breast cancer risk [28], whereas high WC prophesied a non-significant increase in breast cancer incidence in young women [14]. By contrast, in further studies, body fat distribution, such as waist circumference had no defining role in the establishment of insulin resistance or premenopausal breast cancer risk [2,29,32].

Magnetic resonance imaging (MRI) was used to quantify separately the mass of visceral and subcutaneous abdominal fat depositions in obese adolescent girls [38]. Mass of visceral fat was highly correlated with basal insulin secretion, stimulated insulin secretion and insulin resistance. By contrast, WHR value or abdominal subcutaneous fat mass measured by MRI did not show close correlation with the quantified indicators of insulin resistance.

In conclusion, neither BMI nor circumference measurement may discern the indifferent abdominal subcutaneous and the dangerous visceral fat deposition, which explains the highly controversial results regarding correlations between obesity grade and breast cancer risk.

Age-Related Role of Obesity in the Prediction of Breast Cancer Risk

Defining age for the initiation of obesity-associated breast cancer risk is also under debate. Literary data suggest key ages; such as 5, 10, 12, 18 or 20 years, when obesity would determine the breast cancer risk for premenopausal period or for the whole life of patients [4,5,16,26,39,40].

Some studies suppose a definite key age; for example 10 years when breast cancer "protective" obesity turns to harmful between ages 10 and 20 years as a prediction of elevated breast cancer risk in premenopausal phase [41]. Moreover, fatness in childhood was found to be associated with decreased breast cancer risk even in postmenopausal women [40]. Others postulate that only teenager obesity is protective for premenopausal breast cancer initiation but if it is persistent after teenage years than may be replaced by an increased risk for postmenopausal breast cancer [42]. Nevertheless, to find a key age in young girls when obesity turns from cancer protective to cancer promoting agent seemed to be unsuccessful.

In a prospective study in Japan high BMI at 20 years of age seemed to exhibit protective effect for breast cancer risk disregarding the menopausal status and current BMI at tumor diagnosis. In conclusion this postpubertal year was regarded as crucial age for obesity associated cancer prevention [4].

Uncertainty concerning the exact time of tumor initiation proposes a strict distinction between earlier and current obesity. Earlier visceral obesity in puberty and in young ages means a severe danger for insulin resistance and disturbed hormonal equilibrium [43]; however, it may or may not involve cancer initiation. Onset of cancer development may require longer exposition time for harmful systemic disorders; such as visceral obesity and may be counteracted or accelerated by further diverse effects.

Studies reporting on the causal role of current obesity in the year of breast cancer diagnosis cannot estimate the fatness in the unknown year of tumor initiation. Actual BMI and subsequent weight gain were not associated with increased risk among premenopausal women, but predicted increased risk among postmenopausal cases [4]. These results strengthen the lower obesity associated breast cancer risk among young women as compared with postmenopausal cases but don't justify the protective effect of obesity in young cases. Current obesity in the year of tumor diagnosis rather suggests a more rapid progression of tumor and a worse outcome of disease. Actual obesity was an independent prognostic factor for distant metastases and for death in breast cancer cases and was associated with more advanced stages at tumor diagnosis and poorly differentiated grade of cancers [44,45].

Long and unpredictable latency between tumor initiation and clinical tumor diagnosis perfectly disqualifies the strict distinction between pre- and postmenopausal breast cancer cases [46]. A tumor, initiated about at age of 30 years in an obese woman may be clinically manifested both in pre- and postmenopausal period, depending on the rapidity of cancer progression and on the year of menopause.

Dynamism of fatness seems also to be a disturbing factor in obesity studies. A fat adolescent girl may grow to a lean woman and if cancer could not initiate in the obese period of puberty the registered data of body fatness become worthless. By contrast, a lean adolescent girl may become fat young women after childbearing. Correlations between self-reported weight gain, weight loss and breast cancer initiation have also restricted values. In young women weight loss since 18 years did not increase and weight gain did not decrease the risk of breast cancer [47].

After menopause the estimation of adiposity associated breast cancer risk is much simpler. In postmenopausal estrogen deficient obese cases the regional distribution of fat near uniformly affects the visceral region and the increasing prevalence of insulin resistance by years after menopause is well-known [36,37]. Recently, visceral adiposity and the associated high circulating level of insulin and insulin-like growth factors were found to show direct correlation with postmenopausal breast cancer risk independent of serum estrogen level [48]. In older women, never using HRT, the uniformity of obesity associated dangerous metabolic alterations results in strong direct association between adiposity and breast cancer risk [6,30,33]. Studies finding no close association between obesity and postmenopausal breast cancer risk are extremely rare. In a study in Switzerland the low prevalence of overweight and obesity in Swiss population may explain the missing correlation between body fatness and breast cancer risk [27].

Effects of Reproductive Data and Menstrual Factors on Obesity-Associated Breast Cancer Risk

According to the majority of literary data, in premenopausal cases, obesity is associated with decreased circulatory estrogen level [7]. Obesity may confer irregular menstrual cycles, anovulation, infertility and reduced response to fertility treatment in premenopausal women [16]. Nevertheless, anovulatory disorders might also occur in lean young girls without adiposity and even regular menstrual cycles are not the obvious signs of normal ovulatory activity [49]. These diverse associations may explain the fairly controversial findings on correlations between obesity associated anovulatory infertility and breast cancer risk.

Nulliparity may presumably be associated with ovulatory disorders in the majority of cases and there are studies, which equivocally exhibited increased prevalence of breast cancer in nulliparous women [50,51]. Furthermore, coexistence of nulliparity and overweight may amplify each other's effect on increasing breast cancer risk having strong synergism [50] Delayed childbearing proved to be a risk factor of breast cancer among older premenopausal women as well [18,52], which may also be associated with fertility disorders. High breast cancer risk in correlation with nulliparity and delayed first birth are well documented and these results suggest an important role of defective estrogen synthesis and anovulatory disorders in mammary carcinogenesis.

By contrast, many authors presume that either exogenous or endogenous elevated estrogen level may induce mammary carcinogenesis [53,54,55]. Based on this concept, insufficient ovarian estrogen production and a decreased cumulative number of ovulations was presumed to be protective for breast cancer risk [56,57] . Even the physiologic ovulatory peak of circulatory estradiol level during menstrual cycle emerged as dangerous cancer risk. This preconception suggested that ovulation, which is the most important initial step of reproduction endangers the somatic health and life of women.

In a prospective study anovulatory infertility was associated with decreased breast cancer incidence. Surprisingly, greatest reduction in breast cancer incidence was found among those infertile women who underwent to high dose estrogen treatment as ovulation induction therapy [58]. By contrast, a further study of the same working group in the same year established that other factors than anovulatory disorders may be protective against breast cancer risk in obese young women [26].

Menstrual cycle characteristics such as the disorders of cycles, age at menarche and age at menopause have long been hypothesized to affect the incidence of breast cancer.

Results of cohort and case-control studies exhibit inconsistent data concerning the associations of menstrual disorders and breast cancer incidence. Some investigators found an increased breast cancer incidence in women with long menstrual cycles [59,60] others found no associations [61,62,63] or by contrast, a decreased risk [64]. In a large study, in women having long cycles the risk of breast cancer was increased, whereas, in those whose cycle was estimated to be irregular, the risk was reduced [65]! This latter finding was strengthened by a prospective study, which resulted in a significantly reduced risk of breast cancer in women with irregular cycles at ages 41-46 years [57].

Strongly controversial correlations between irregular menstrual cycles and breast cancer risk yielded a constrained presumption; either a lesser or a greater cumulative number of ovulatory cycles mean increased breast cancer risk [59].

In the Nurses' Health Study II, the authors tried to define a key age period to prophesy premenopausal breast cancer risk based on menstrual characteristics. Among women with long or irregular menstrual cycles at ages 18 to 22 years, only young premenopausal women below 40 years experienced a decreased risk of breast cancer as compared with cases having normal cycles [66]. These correlations suggest that determinant hormonal defects at ages 18 to 22 definitely could prophesy lower breast cancer incidence restricted to young premenopausal cases.

Controversial associations between breast cancer risk and anovulatory menstrual disorders could not justify the beneficial impact of defective estrogen synthesis and low circulatory estrogen level.

Age at menarche has been supported to be closely correlated with breast cancer risk but results concerning these associations are fairly controversial as well. Decreased breast cancer risk in women with late menarcheal age of 15 years or more as compared those with menarche at age 13 was established by a population based study [62]. This relation was especially strong for premenopausal breast cancer cases as opposed to postmenopausals. Similarly, later menarche and body fatness at age 10 years were found to be closely associated with decreased risk for premenopausal breast cancer [41].

Breast cancer risk seemed to be increased by early menarche [56]. However, early age at menarche could not significantly modify the risk for premenopausal breast cancer neither in Atlanta nor in Spain [18,67].

Age at menopause defines preferentially the length of reproductive life. As a preconception, early menopause was suspected as breast cancer protective, whereas late menopause as tumor promoting factor. Early menopause, either natural or surgical was shown to be associated with decreased breast cancer risk. Surgical menopause before 40 conferred the strongest cancer protective effect [62]. Conversely, as a milestone in prospective breast tumor investigations, long lasting breast cancer protective capacity of estrogen treatment was observed in uniformly endangered hysterectomised postmenopausal women [68,69]. These results justified the advantageous effect of estrogen replacement against breast cancer in highly endangered hysterectomised women [46].

Late menopause was not associated with increased breast cancer risk in a large population based case-control study [62]. By contrast, a review of associations between hormones and cancer risk established that cancers in the highly hormone responsive organs (endometrial, ovarian and breast cancers) exhibit increased incidence rate with late menopause [56]. These contradictory results concerning the correlations between age at menopause and breast cancer risk require revision.

Effects of Exogenous Hormone Treatment on Breast Cancer Risk

Oral contraceptive use is a long lasting hormone treatment and there are controversial data concerning its predictive value for breast cancer. Among young cases, below 35 years, recent use of oral contraceptives was regarded as significant breast cancer predictor [18]. Contraceptive use at early ages or of long duration was reported having particular signify-cance in the etiology of early onset breast cancer [52]. By contrast, oral contraceptive use was established as decreasing factor for breast, endometrial and ovarian cancer incidence [56,70]. These latter findings were explained by the assumption that contraception is advantageous against cancer risk by reducing the number of ovulations. Authors devoted to the principle of the carcinogenic capacity of estrogen suggest that multiparity have cancer protective effect by lowering the lifetime cumulated number of ovulations. Multiparity and risk for malignancies exhibit an inverse relationship indeed [71,72,73] even in cases of highly hormone responsive tumors; such as breast, endometrial and ovarian cancer [56,74].

HRT use has highly controversial associations with breast cancer risk. Till now, the carcinogenic capacity of postmenopausal estrogen therapy was a prevailing concept [75,76]. Recently, there are overwhelming results supporting the cancer protective capacity of postmenopausal estrogen treatment not only for moderately hormone responsive organs but also for female breast [68,69,77,78,79,80,81,82,83,84,85]. Results of these recent studies prepare an earthquake regarding the concept of mammary carcinogenesis. Increasing number of investigations exhibits the benefit of HRT for women as it reduces breast cancer risk and other chronic diseases after menopause [69,85,86,87,88].

HRT decreases the accumulation of central fatty tissue in obese postmenopausal women and provides long term metabolic and health benefits for them [48,89]. HRT use equivocally attenuates the obesity-associated breast cancer risk [14,15,86,90] similarly like does it the preserved circulatory estrogen level in fat premenopausal women. In conclusion, estrogen treatment in postmenopausal women decreases the severity of insulin resistance and obesity associated breast cancer incidence as well.

Obesity Related Metabolic and Hormonal Disorders as Mediators of Breast Cancer Risk

Obesity and breast cancer risk are not in direct correlation, rather adiposity associated complex systemic alterations may confer increased breast cancer incidence. This indirect association between obesity and breast cancer risk may explain many debated controversies concerning the presumed protective effect of obesity for breast cancer in young women. Moreover, mammary carcinogenesis exhibits multicausal nature influenced by diverse exogenous and systemic factors being independent of obesity.

Obesity itself is a multifaceted disorder and the associated metabolic and hormonal disturbances are not uniform, particularly in young women in their reproductive period. Literary data reflect controversial correlations between the *extent and type of obesity* and the risk of breast cancer. Some studies could find close correlations between body fat distribution and breast cancer risk, particularly in young cases [14,28,33]. Further authors could not justify that fatty tissue distribution would play an important role in the overall incidence of premenopausal breast cancer [29]. Nevertheless, neither body mass index nor abdominal circumference measurements could equivocally define the severity of insulin resistance [38], so their value in prophesying the premenopausal risk of breast cancer did not prove to be reliable.

Diverse distributions of fat deposition and their different relations to insulin resistance and estrogen deficiency might be important factors by which an indirect, low obesity associated breast cancer risk can be justified in premenopausal cases. Inconsistent clinical results yielded the misleading concept concerning the protective effect of fatness for breast cancer.

Studies searching a *key age in children* to determine the year of the presumed breast cancer protective effect of obesity yielded fairly controversial results. Nevertheless, obesity may not be protective even in children. Childhood obesity is diversely associated with insulin resistance and hyperinsulinemia conferring different risk for chronic diseases and cancer in the adult life [91]. Many factors of metabolic syndrome, such as elevated glucose level, hypertension, high triglyceride and low HDL-cholesterol level even type-2 diabetes might occur in these young prepubertal obese cases [92].

Period of puberty with extreme somatic growth and explosion-like sexual development means a great challenge for whole metabolic and hormonal systems. Danger of insulin resistance increases with adolescence even in cases with normal body weight [93]. Childhood obesity becomes a more serious health risk in puberty and will confer higher increase in insulin resistance and hyperinsulinism than in normal weight children [38]. In obese adolescent, increased insulin resistance does not return to prepubertal values at the end of puberty and means a high risk for adult metabolic syndrome, type-2 diabetes and their complications [92,94].

In adolescent girls, obesity associated metabolic storms are related to abnormal ovarian sexual steroidgenesis as well, resulting in excessive androgen production and they exhibit greater frequency of anovulatory cycles [5,95]. Studies on endocrine determinants of fertility supported that high serum androgen concentrations in puberty are preserved into adulthood and are reflected by defective fertility patterns at least until 30 years of age [96]. This observation may be in concordance with the increased premenopausal breast cancer risk of delayed first childbearing [18,52].

Obesity is never cancer protective it always endangers the health of women. Androgen excess, defective estrogen synthesis and insulin resistance are obesity associated disorders conferring high breast cancer risk in the whole life of obese adolescent girl [95,97]. Consequently, developing systemic alterations in puberty and young age might be really defining for the breast cancer risk of obese girls, but they are not protective, rather highly dangerous.

Equilibrium of sexual hormone production and the development of regular cycles are prerequisites not only for reproduction but also for somatic health in women [19,20,46]Biologically relevant roles of estrogen and its receptor signals represent a mean of high integration between reproductive functions and metabolic balance serving individual's survival [98]. Pathological alterations, such as obesity, endangering both the fertility and survival of women might not be protective for cancer initiation either in pre- or postmenopausal cases.

Anovulatory infertility and irregular menstrual cycles might be in close correlation with breast cancer risk even without obesity. In premenopausal women with polycystic ovarian syndrome (PCOS) the coexistence of infertility and insulin resistance means common risk for the cancers of highly hormone dependent breast, endometrium and ovary [99]. Mortality data of infertile women with PCOS were examined in a long-term follow up study in the UK and breast cancer was the most common cause of deaths among them [100]. In a further study, nulliparity, irregular menstrual cycles, diabetes and hypertension were strongly associated with endometrial cancer risk and in addition a high incidence of synchronous primary ovarian cancers were also observed in premenopausal women [101].

Ambiguous results concerning the correlation between obesity associated hormonal disturbances and breast cancer risk may be explained by the facts that infertility and anovulation are not always associated with either clinically observed menstrual disorders or obesity. Among symptom-free lean insulin resistant girls laboratory findings of hyperinsulinemia and excessive androgen concentration may reveal the occult anovulatory cycles [49].

How can we explain the predilection for increased breast, endometrial and ovarian cancer risk in women with fertility disorders even without obesity? In these anovulatory premenopausal cases, circulating female sexual steroid levels are slightly or moderately decreased associated with excessive androgen concentrations and hyperinsulinism. These disorders confer particular cancer risk for highly estrogen dependent organs, such as female breast [19,20,46].

Parity of women reflects their fertility in the majority of cases. Nulliparity and delayed first childbearing are near equivocally associated with increased breast cancer risk [18,50,51,52] and they supposedly are predominantly in correlation with defective estrogen synthesis and fertility disorders.

On the contrary, breast cancer protective effect of multiparity was justified in several studies [56,74]. Increased estrogen level in pregnancy and a healthy equilibrium of female sexual steroid production associated with good fertility may have tumor protective effect not only for female breast but also for other organs [19,46]. Nevertheless, pregnancy equivalent, high female sexual hormone treatment could prevent even chemically induced mammary carcinogenesis in female Lewis rats [102].

Counteraction between Obesity Associated Insulin Resistance and Protective Circulatory Estrogen Level

In *premenopausal women* combat between obesity associated insulin resistance and the counteracting exogenous and systemic protective factors, such as circulatory estrogen level will decide the initiation of breast cancer [19,103]. In premenopausal obese cases milder insulin resistance may be counteracted by slightly altered but essentially preserved hormonal cycle and yet sufficient estradiol level. By contrast, if premenopausal obesity confers a severe form of insulin resistance, the beneficial but defective estrogen synthesis will be defeated and cancer may develop. Both hyperinsulinism and androgen excess associated with insulin resistance are strong carcinogenic injuries without sufficient available circulatory estrogen level. In conclusion, in obese premenopausal women their preserved estrogen level confers protective effect for breast cancer instead of obesity and the associated insulin resistance.

Obese postmenopausal women without hormone treatment have high breast cancer risk, whereas HRT use equivocally reduces their breast cancer incidence [13,14,15]. A great challenge to explain the beneficial anticancer impact of HRT in postmenopausal women with high BMI based on the belief that they have excessive circulatory estrogen level [1]. To solve this contradiction, some authors assumed that other mediators, such as insulin and insulin-like growth factors may confer obesity associated breast cancer risk, rather than estrogen [5,48].

Postmenopausal obese women, never using HRT are insulin resistant. Moreover, ageing after menopause is an increasing risk as it is associated with a continuously deepening estrogen loss and parallel increasing insulin resistance [36,37]. In old obese women, struggle between the harmful components of insulin resistance and the low level of protective female sexual steroids will be frequently finished by cancer initiation. These correlations explain the high breast cancer risk of obese postmenopausal women without hormone treatment.

In obese postmenopausal women using HRT the protective effect of estrogen substitution may counteract to obesity associated insulin resistance [48,89] and their breast cancer risk decreases. Their hormonal and metabolic equilibrium becomes similar to that of obese young women with preserved circulatory estrogen levels. Estradiol substitution increases insulin sensitivity [104] yields favorable changes in plasma lipid levels [105] and by its anti-obesity effect decreases the accumulation of visceral fat deposition [89]. All these impacts justify the anticancer capacity of HRT after menopause.

In recent experimental studies estrogen exhibited protective effect against breast cancer in obese animals. In ovariectomized female mice, estrogen substitution triggered the loss of body fat, enhanced insulin sensitivity and suppressed the growth of subcutaneously transplanted mammary tumors [106]. Equilibrium of circulating female sexual steroid levels and fertility decreases during women's life. Ability for conception is on the top in young women under 30 years of age and in the fourth decade it continuously declines suggesting decreasing fertility and hormonal activity even in the premenopausal period [107]. Menopause at 50-51years means a sudden break in ovarian estrogen production and confers further steep decline in circulating hormone level. In postmenopausal phase a compensatory estrogen production of tissues having high estrogen demand, such as female breast, seems to be an ability to preserve their integrity and health but it is not always satisfying and never excessive [98]. New approach to measure estrogen levels and metabolism by highly sensitive methods may change the earlier results of estrogen studies in postmenopausal cases [108,109]. Comparison of this new method with classic indirect radioimmunoassay and enzyme-linked immunosorbent assay showed consistently lower estrogen concentrations as compared with earlier data, especially at the low levels of postmenopausal women. This new method can be useful to access the clinical significance of decrease in serum estrogen levels after menopause. Continuous decline in circulating estrogens during women's life may reveal the cause of increase in breast cancer incidence without any ambiguous interaction between obesity and menopausal status. Obesity by its associated deteriorating alterations increases breast cancer risk both in premenopausal and postmenopausal phases during the whole life of women. Correlations between adiposity and breast cancer risk within different age categories justified that breast cancer risk is lowest below 35 and highest above 65 years of age [6]. These data seem to justify that the two poles of life exhibit greatest differences in breast cancer incidence.

Conclusion

Obesity-associated metabolic and hormonal disorders confer high breast cancer risk during the whole life of women. Multicausal nature of breast cancer and the complexity of its risk factors may explain the controversial inconsistent results gained on indirect correlations between obesity and breast cancer risk.Defense mechanisms against obesity-associated breast cancer initiation exhibit parallelism in pre- and postmenopausal cases. In premenopause, relatively preserved circulatory estrogen level, in postmenopausal women, hormone replacement therapy represents protective anticancer capacity. These correlations explain the lower breast cancer risk of obese young women as compared with fat older cases. Moreover, these aspects illuminate the beneficial, decreased breast cancer risk in obese postmenopausal cases with hormone treatment as compared with those never using HRT.

Recognition of correlations between continuous decrease in circulatory estrogen levels and increase in breast cancer incidence during women's life means advance in understanding breast cancer etiology and promotes possibilities for primary tumor prevention.

References

[1] Rose D. P., Vona-Davis L.: Interaction between menopausal status and obesity in affecting breast cancer risk. *Maturitas* 66:33-38, 2010.

[2] Franceschi S., Favero A., La Vecchia C., Barón A. E., Negri E., Dal Maso L., Giacosa A et al.: Body size indices and breast cancer risk before and after menopause. *Int. J. Cancer* 67:181-6, 1966.

[3] Ursin G., Longnecker M. P., Haile R. W., Greenland S.: A meta-analysis of body mass index and risk of premenopausal breast cancer. *Epidemiology* 6:137-141, 1995.

[4] Suzuki R., Iwasaki M., Inoue M., Sasazuki S., Sawada N., Yamaji T., Shimazu T., Tsugane S.: Body weight at age 20 years, subsequent weight change and breast cancer risk defined by estrogen and progesterone receptor status – the Japan public health center-based study. *Int. J. Cancer* 129:1214-24, 2011.

[5] Baer H. J., Tworoger S. S., Hankinson S. E., Willett W. C.: Body fatness at young ages and risk of breast cancer throughout life. *Am. J. Epidemiol.* 171:1183-94, 2010.

[6] La Vecchia C., Negri E., Franceschi S. et al: Body mass index and postmenopausal breast cancer: an age specific analysis. *Br. J. Cancer* 75:441-444, 1997.

[7] Potischman N., Swanson C. A., Siiteri P., Hoover R. N.: Reveal of relation between body mass and endogenous estrogen concentrations with menopausal status. *J. Natl. Cancer Inst.* 88:756-758, 1996.

[8] Rose D. P., Vona-Davis I.: Influence of obesity on breast cancer receptor status and prognosis. *Expert Rev. Anticancer Ther.* 9:1091-101, 2009.

[9] Vona-Davis I., Howard-McNatt M., Rose D. P.: Adiposity, type-2 diabetes and the metabolic syndrome in breast cancer. *Obes. Rev.* 8:395-408, 2007.

[10] International Agency for Research on Cancer: Monographs on the evaluation of carcinogenic risks to humans: hormonal contraception and postmenopausal hormone therapy. *I. A. R. C.*, Lyon, France, vol. 72, 1999.

[11] Key T., ApplebyP., Barnes I., Reeves G.: Endogenous hormones and Breast Cancer Collaborative Group.Endogenous sex hormones and breast cancer in postmenopausal women: reanalysis of nine prospective studies. *J. Natl. Cancer Inst.* 94:606-616, 2002.

[12] Lahmann P. H., Hoffmann K., Allen N. et al.: Body size and breast cancer risk: findings from the European Prospective Investigation into Cancer and Nutrition (E. P. I. C.). *Int. J. Cancer* 111:762-771, 2004.

[13] Howell A., Chapman M., Harvie M.: Energy restriction for breast cancer prevention. *Recent Results Cancer Res.* 181:97-111, 2009.

[14] Huang Z., Willett W. C., Colditz G. A. et al.: Waist circumference, waist:hip ratio, and risk of breast cancer in the Nurses' Health Study. *Am. J. Epidemiol.* 150:1316-24, 1999.

[15] Morimoto L. M., White E., Chen Z. et al: Obesity, body size and risk of postmenopausal breast cancer: the Women's Health Initiative (United States). *Cancer Causes Control* 13:41-51, 2002.

[16] Zain M. M., Norman R. J.: Impact of obesity on female fertility and fertility treatment. *Womens Health* (Lond Engl.) 4:183-94, 2008.

[17] Stephenson G. D., Rose D. P.: Breast cancer and obesity: an update. *Nutr. Cancer* 45:1-16, 2003.

[18] Althuis M. D., Brogan D. D., Coates R. J., Gammon M. D., Malone K. E., Schoenberg J. B., Brinton L. A.: Breast cancers among very young premenopausal women (United States). *Cancer Causes Control* 14:151-60, 2003.

[19] Suba Z.: Interplay between insulin resistance and estrogen deficiency as co-activators in carcinogenesis. *Pathol. Oncol. Res*., 18:123-133, 2012.

[20] Suba Z.: Insulin resistance, estrogen deficiency and cancer risk. *In: Estrogen versus Cancer*. Chapter 7. pp. 127-146. Nova Science Publishers Inc. New York, 2009.

[21] SubaZs.: Obesity and risk for salivary gland tumors. Chapter 3. pp. 71-86. Ramonde P. R. and Fochas E. H. eds.: *Obesity and cancer research*. Nova Science Publishers Inc. New York, 2009.

[22] SubaZs.: Correlations between obesity and risk for salivary gland tumors. *Cancer Res. J*. 3:55-68, 2009.

[23] Björntorp P.: The regulation of adipose tissue distribution in humans. *Int. J. Obes. Relat. Metab. Disord*. 20:291-302, 1996.

[24] Leitzmann M. F., Moore S. C., Peters T. M., Lacey J. V. Jr., Schatzkin A., Schairer C., Brinton L. A., Albanes D.: Prospective study of physical activity and risk of postmenopausal breast cancer. *Breast Cancer Res*. 10:R92, 2008.

[25] Teras L. R., Goodman M., Patel A. V., Diver W. R., Flanders W. D., Feigelson H. S.: Weight loss and postmenopausal breast cancer in a prospective cohort of overweight and obese women. *Cancer Causes Control*. 22:573-579, 2011.

[26] Michels K. B., Terry K. L., Willett W. C.: Longitudinal study on the role of body size in premenopausal breast cancer. *Arch. Intern. Med*. 166:2395-402, 2006.

[27] Eichholzer M., Schmid S. M., Bovey F., Jordan P., Rohrmann S., Huang D. J., Rochlitz C., Güth U.: Impact of overweight and obesity on postmenopausal breast cancer: analysis of 20-year data from Switzerland. *Arch. Gynecol. Obstetrics*. Aug. 4 [Epub ahead of print] 2011.

[28] Fagherazzi G., Chabbert-Buffet N., Fabre A., Guillas G., Boutron-Ruault M. C., Mesrine S., Clavel-Chapelon F.: Hip circumference is associated with the risk of premenopausal ER-/PR- breast cancer. *Int. J. Obes*. (Lond.) 36:431-9, 2012.

[29] Harris H. R., Willett W. C., Terry K. L., Michels K. B.: Body fat distribution and risk of premenopausal breast cancer in the Nurses' Health Study II. *J. Natl. Cancer Inst*. 103:273-8, 2011.

[30] Phipps A. I., Chlebowski R. T., Prentice R., McTiernan A., Stefanick M. L., Wactawski-Wende J., Kuller L. H., Adams-Campbell L. L., Lane D., Vitolins M., Kabat G. C., Rohan T. E., Li C. I.: Body size, physical activity, and risk of triple-negative and estrogen receptor-positive breast cancer. *Cancer Epidemiol. Biomarkers Prev*. 20:454-63, 2011.

[31] Sun C. A., Wu M. H., Chu C. H., Chou Y. C., Hsu G. C., Yang T., Chou W. Y., Yu C. P., Yu J. C.: Adipocytokine resistin and breast cancer risk. *Breast Cancer Res. Treat* 123:869-76, 2010.

[32] Kotlyarevska K., Wolfgram P., Lee J. M.: Is waist circumference a better predictor of insulin resistance than body mass index in US adolescents? *J. Adolesc. Health* 49:330-3, 2011.

[33] Sonnenschein E., Toniolo P., Terry M. B., Bruning P. F., Kato I., Koenig K. L., Shore R. E.: Body fat distribution and obesity in pre- and postmenopausal breast cancer. *Int. J. Epidemiol*. 28:1026-31, 1999.

[34] Page J. H., Rexrode K. M., Hu F., Albert C. M., Chae C. U., Manson J. E.: Waist-height ratio as a predictor of coronary heart disease among women. *Epidemiology* 20:361-6, 2009.

[35] Poehlman, E.T., Toth, M.J., Gardner, A.W.: Changes in energy balance and body composition at menopause. *Ann. Intern. Med.*123:673-675, 1995.

[36] Schneider J. G., Tompkins C., Blumenthal R. S., Mora S.: The metabolic syndrome in women. *Cardiol. Rev.* 14:286-291, 2006.

[37] Wu, Sh.I., Chou, P., Tsai, Sh.T.: The impact of years since menopause on the development of impaired glucose tolerance. *J. Clin. Epidemiol.* 54:117-120, 2001.

[38] Caprio S., Hyman L. D., Limb C., McCarthy S., Lange R., Sherwin R. S., Shulman G., Tamborlane V. V. V.: Central adiposity and its metabolic correlates in obese adolescent girls. *Am. J. Physiol.* 269:E118-26, 1995.

[39] Poole E. M., Tworoger S. S., Hankinson S. E., Schernhammer E. S., Pollak M. N., Baer H. J.: Body size in early life and adult levels of insulin-like growth factor 1 and insulin-like growth factor binding protein 3. *Am. J. Epidemiol.* 174:642-51, 2011.

[40] Bardia A., Vachon C. M., Olson J. E., Vierkant R. A., Wang A. H., Hartmann L. L., Sellers T. A., Cerhan J. R.: Relative weight at age 12 and risk of postmenopausal breast cancer. *Cancer Epidemiol. Biomarkers Prev.* 17:374-378, 2008.

[41] Berkey C. S., Frazier A. L., Gardner J. D., Colditz G. A.: Adolescence and breast carcinoma risk. *Cancer* 85:2400-2409, 1999.

[42] Stoll B. A.: Teenage obesity in relation to breast cancer risk. *Int. J. Obes. Relat. Metab. Disord.* 22:1035-1040, 1998.

[43] Colditz G. A., Frazier A. L.: Models of breast cancer show that risk is set by events of early life: prevention efforts must shift focus. *Cancer Epidemiol. Biomarkers Prev.* 4:567-71, 1995.

[44] Ewertz M., Jensen M. B., Gunnarsdóttir K. Á., Jakobson E. H., Nielsen D., Stenbygaard L. E., Tange U. B., Cold S.: Effect of obesity on prognosis after early-stage breast cancer. *J. Clin. Oncol.* 29:25-31, 2011.

[45] Stark A., Stahl M. S., Kirchner H. L., Krum S., Prichard J., Evans J.: Body maass index at the time of diagnosis and the risk of advanced stages and poorly differentiated cancers of the breast: findings from a case-control study. *Int. J. Obes.* (Lond.) 34:1381-6, 2010.

[46] Suba Z.: Common soil of smoking-associated and hormone-related cancers: estrogen deficiency. *Oncol. Rev.* 4:73-87, 2010.

[47] Michels K. B., Terry K. L., Eliassen A. H., Hankinson S. E., Willett W. C.:Adult weight change and incidence of premenopausal breast cancer. *Int. J. Cancer* 130:902-9 2012.

[48] Gunter J. M., Hoover D. R., Yu H. et al.: Insulin, insulin-like growth factor and risk of breast cancer in postmenopausal women. *J. Natl. Cancer Inst.* 101:48-60, 2009.

[49] Bloomgarden Z. T. Second World Congress on the Insulin Resistance Syndrome: Mediators, pediatric insulin resistance, the polycystic ovary syndrome, and malignancy. *Diabetes Care* 28:1821-1830, 2005.

[50] Opdahl S., Alsaker M. D., Janszky I., Romundstad P. R., Vatten L. J.: Joint effect of nulliparity and other breast cancer risk factors. *Br. J. Cancer* 105:731-6, 2011.

[51] Newcomb P. A., Trentham-Dietz A., Hampton J. M., Egan K. M., Titus-Ernstoff L., Warren Andersen S., Greenberg E. R., Willett W. C.: Late age at full term birth is strongly associated with lobular breast cancer.*Cancer* 117:1946-56, 2011.

[52] Velentgas P., Daling J. R.: Risk factors for breast cancer in younger women. *J. Natl. Cancer Inst. Monogr.* 16:15-24, 1994.

[53] Berrino F., Muti P., Micheli A., Bolelli G., Krogh V., Sciajno R. et al.: Serum sex hormon levels after menopause and subsequent breast cancer. *J. Natl. Cancer Inst.* 88:291-296, 1996.

[54] Feigelson H. S., Henderson B. E.: Estrogens and breast cancer. *Carcinogenesis* 17:2279-2284, 1996.

[55] Toniolo P. G., Levitz M., Zeleniuch-Jacquotte A., Banerjee S., Koenig K. L., Shore R. E., Strax P., Pasternak B. S.: A prospective study of endogenous estrogens and breast cancer in post-menopausal women. *J. Natl. Cancer Inst.* 87:190-197, 1995.

[56] Key T. J.: Hormones and cancer in humans. *Mutat. Res.* 333:59-67, 1995.

[57] denTonkelaar I., de Waard F.: Regularity and length of menstrual cycles in women aged 41-46 in relation to breast cancer risk: results from the DOM-project. *Breast Cancer Res. Treat.* 38:253-8, 1996.

[58] Terry K. L., Willett W. C., Rich-Edwards J. W., Michels K. B.: A prospective study of infertility due to ovulatory disorders, ovulation induction, and incidence of breast cancer. *Arch. Intern. Med.* 166:2484-9, 2006.

[59] Whelan E. A., Sandler D. P., Root J. L., Smith K. R., Weinberg C. R.: Menstrual cycle patterns and risk of breast cancer. *Am. J. Epidemiol.* 140:1081-90, 1994.

[60] Yuan J. M., Yu M. C., Ross R. K., Gao Y. T., Henderson B. E.: Risk factors for breast cancer in Chinese women in Shanghai. *Cancer Res.* 48:1949-53, 1988.

[61] Clavel-Chapelon F.: Cumulative number of menstrual cycles and breast cancer risk: results from the E3N cohort study of French women. *Cancer Causes Control.* 13:831-8, 2002.

[62] Titus-Ernstoff L., Longnecker M. P., Newcomb P. A., Dain B., Greenberg E. R., Mittendorf R., Stampfer M., Willett W.: Menstrual factors in relation to breast cancer risk. *Cancer Epidemiol. Biomarkers Prev.* 7:783-789, 1998.

[63] Gao Y. T., Shu X. O., Dai Q. et al.: Association of menstrual and reproductive factors with breast cancer risk: results from the Sanghai Breast Cancer Study. *Int. J. Cancer* 87:295-300, 2000.

[64] Wu A. H., Ziegler R. G., Pike M. C. et al.: Menstrual and reproductive factors and risk of breast cancer in Asian-Americans. *Br. J. Cancer* 73:680-686, 1996.

[65] Parazzini F., La Vecchia C., Negri E., Franceschi S., Tozzi L.: Lifelong menstrual patterns and risk of breast cancer. *Oncology* 50:222-25, 1993.

[66] Terry K. L., Willett W. C., Rich-Edwards J. W., Hunter D. J., Michels K. B.: Menstrual cycle characteristics and incidence of premenopausal breast cancer. *Cancer Epidemiol. Biomarkers Prev.* 14:1509-13, 2005.

[67] Mendosa N.,Galliano D., Salamanca A., Castro J. E., Mozas J., Sánchez-Borrego R., Quereda F., Vázquez F., Martinez-Astorquiza T.: Lowering the age at menarche and risk of early menarche in a population of Spanish postmenopausal women during the past two decades. *Menopause Int.* 16:111-4, 2010.

[68] Anderson G. L., Limacher M., Assaf A. R., Bassford T., Beresford S. A., Black H., Bonds D. et al.: Women's Health Intitative Steering Committee. Effects of conjugated equine estrogen in postmenopausal women with hysterectomy: the Women's Health Intitative randomized controlled trial. *J. A. M. A.* 291:1701-1712, 2004.
[69] LaCroix A. Z., Chlebowski R. T., Manson J. E., Aragaki A. K., Johnson K. C., Martin L. et al.: Health outcomes after stopping conjugated equine estrogens among postmenopausal women with prior hysterectomy. A randomized controlled trial. *J. A. M. A.* 305:305-1314, 2011.
[70] La Vecchia C., Franceschi S.: Oral contraceptives and ovarian cancer. *Eur. J. Cancer Prev.* 8:297-304, 1999.
[71] Wolpert B. J., Amr S., Ezzat S., Saleh D., Gouda I., Loay I. et al.: Estrogen exposure and bladder cancer risk in Egyptian women. *Maturitas* 67:353-357, 2010.
[72] Teras L. R., Patel A. V., Rodriguez C., Thun M. J., Calle E. E.: Parity, other reproductive factors, and risk of pancreatic cancer mortality in a large cohort of US women. *Cancer Causes and Control* 16:1035-40, 2005.
[73] Bosetti C., Negri E., Franceschi S., Conti E., Levi F., Tomei F., La Vecchia C.: Risk factors for oral and pharyngeal cancer in women: a study from Italy and Switzerland. *Br. J. Cancer* 82:204-207, 2000.
[74] Britt K., Ashworth A., Smalley M.: Pregnancy and the risk of breast cancer. *Endocrine-Related Cancer* 14:907-933, 2007.
[75] Diamanti-Kandarakis E.: Hormone replacement therapy and risk of malignancy. *Current Opin. Obstet Gynecol.* 16:73-78, 2004.
[76] Rossouw J.E., Anderson G.L., Prentice R.L., La Croix A.Z. et al; Wrighting Group for the Women's Health Initiative Investigators: Risks and benefits of estrogen plus progestin in healthy postmenopausal women: principal results from the Women's Health Initiative randomized controlled trial. *J. A. M. A.* 288:321-333, 2002.
[77] La Vecchia C., Brinton L. A., McTiernan A.: Menopause, hormone replacement therapy and cancer. *Maturitas* 39:97-115, 2001.
[78] La Vecchia C., D'Avanzo B., Franceschi S., Negri E., Parazzini F., Decarli A.: Menstrual and reproductive factors and gastric-cancer in women. *Int. J. Cancer* 59:761-764, 1994.
[79] Olsson H., Bladström A. M., Ingvar C.: Are smoking-associated cancers prevented or postponed in women using hormone replacement therapy? *Obstet. Gynecol.* 102:565-570, 2003.
[80] Gallus S., Bosetti C., Franceschi S., Levi F, Simonato L., Negri E., La Vecchia C.: Oesophageal cancer in women: tobacco, alcohol, nutritional and hormonal factors. *Br. J. Cancer* 85:341-345, 2001.
[81] Camargo M. C., Goto Y., Zabaleta J., Morgan D., Correa P., Rabkin C. S.: Sex hormones, hormonal interventions and gastric cancer risk: A meta-analysis. *Cancer Epidemiol Biomarkers Prev.* Oct. 25 (Epub ahead of print) 2011.
[82] Parazzini F., La Vecchia C., Negri E., Franceschi S., Bolis G.: Case-control study of estrogen replacement therapy and risk of cervical cancer. *Br. Med. J.* 315:85-88, 1997.
[83] Kreuzer M., Gerken M., Heinrich J., Kreienbrock L., Wichmann H. E.: Hormonal factors and risk of lung cancer among women? *Int. J. Epidemiol.* 32:263-271, 2003.

[84] Fernandez E., Gallus S., Bosetti C., Franceschi S., Negri E., La Vecchia C: Hormone replacement therapy and cancer risk: a systematic analysis from a network of case-control studies. *Int. J. Cancer* 105:408-412, 2003.

[85] Ragaz J., Wilson K., Frohlich J., Muraca G., Budlovsky J.: Dual estrogen effects on breast cancer: endogenous estrogen stimulates, exogenous estrogen protects. Further investigation of estrogen chemoprevention is warranted. *Cancer Res.* 70(suppl. 24): 441, 2010.

[86] Howell A., Evans G. D.: Hormone replacement therapy and breast cancer. *Recent Results Cancer Res.* 188:115-24, 2011.

[87] Chlebowski R.T., Anderson G.L.: Changing Concepts: Menopausal hormone therapy and breast cancer. *J. Natl. Cancer Inst.*104:517-27, 2012.

[88] Stevenson J. C., Hodis H. N., Pickar J. H., Lobo R. A.: H. R. T. and breast cancer risk: a realistic perspective. *Climacteric*14:633-6, 2011.

[89] Tchernof A., Calles-Escandon J., Sites C. K., Poehlman E. T.: Menopause, central body fatness and insulin resistance: effects of hormone-replacement therapy. *Coron Artery Dis.* 9:503-11, 1998.

[90] van den Brandt P. A., Spiegelman D., Yaun S. S. et al: Pooled analysis of prospectve cohort studies on height, weight an breast cancer risk. *Am. J. Epidemiol.* 152:514-27, 2000.

[91] Tobisch B., Blatniczky L., Barkai L.: Correlation between insulin resistance and puberty in children with increased cardiometabolic risk. *Orv. Hetil.* 152:1068-74, 2011.

[92] Theintz G.: From obesity to type 2 diabetes in children and adolescents. *Rev. Med. Suisse* 2005;1:477-480, 2005.

[93] Pilia S., Casini M. R., Foschini M. L., Minerba L., Musiu M. C., Marras V., Civolani P., Loche S.: The effect of puberty on insulin resistance in obese children. *J. Endocrinol. Invest* 32:401-5, 2009.

[94] Vanhala M. J., Vanhala P. T., Keinanen-Klukaanniemi S. M. et al.: Relative weight gain and obesity as a child predict metabolic syndrome as an adult. *Int. J. Obes. Relat. Metab. Disord.* 23:656-659, 1999.

[95] Stoll B. A.: Teenage obesity in relation to breast cancer risk. *Int. J. Obes. Relat. Metab. Disord.* 22(11):1035-40, 1998.

[96] Apter D., Vihko R.: Endocrine determinants of fertility: serum androgen concentration during follow-up of adolescents into the third decade of life. *J. Clin. Endocrinol. Metab.* 71:970-974, 1990.

[97] Baer H. J., Colditz G. A., Willett W. C. et al: Adiposity and sex hormones in girls. *Cancer Epidemiol. Biomarkers Prev.* 16:1880-1888, 2007.

[98] Suba Z.: Antiestrogen or estrogen as anticancer drug. Chapter 4. In: Hoffman A. B. (ed): *Sex hormones, Development, Regulation and Disorders.* Nova Science Publishers Inc. New York, 2011.

[99] Gadducci A., Gargini A., Palla E., Fanucchi A., Genazzani A. R.: Polycystic ovary syndrome and gynecological cancers: is there a link? *Gynecol. Endocrinol.* 2005;20:200-208, 2005.

[100] Pierpoint T., McKeigue P. M., Isaacs A. J., Wild S. H., Jacobs H. S.: Mortality of women with polycystic ovary syndrome at long-term follow-up. *J. Clin. Epidemiol.* 51:581-586, 1998.

[101] Soliman P. T., Oh J. C., Schmeler K. M., Sun C. C., Slomovitz B. M., Gershenson D. M., Burke T. W., Lu K. H.: Risk factors for young premenopausal women with endometrial cancer. *Obstet. Gynecol.* 105:575-580, 2005.

[102] Lay Y. C., Hamazaki K., Yoshizawa K., Kawanaka A., Kuwata M., Kanematsu S., Hamazaki T. et al.: Short-term pregnancy hormone treatment of N-methyl-N-nitrosourea-induced mammary carcinogenesis in relation to fatty acid composition of serum phospholipids in female Lewis rats. *In vivo* 24:553-60, 2010.

[103] Suba Z.: Re-evaluation of the epidemiological associations of female sexual steroids and cancer risk. Chapter 6. In: *Estrogen versus Cancer*. Nova Science Publishers Inc. New York, 2009.

[104] Barros R. P. A., Machado U. F., Gustafsson J. A.: Estrogen receptors: new players in diabetes mellitus. *Trends Molecular Med.* 9:425-431, 2006.

[105] Walsh B. W., Schiff I., Rosner B., Greenberg L., Ravinkar V., Sacks F. M.: Effects of postmenopausal estrogen replacement on the concentrations and metabolism of plasma lipoproteins. *New England J. Med.* 1991;325:1196-1204, 1991.

[106] Hong J., Holcomb V. B., Kushiro K., Núnez N. P.: Estrogen inhibits the effects of obesity and alcohol on mammary tumors and fatty liver. *Int. J. Oncol.* 2011;39: 1443-1453, 2011.

[107] Gurtcheff S. E., Klein N. A.: Diminished ovarian reserve and infertility. *Clin. Obstet Gynecol.* 54:666-74, 2011.

[108] Rothman M. S., Carlson N. E., Xu M., Wang C., Swerdloff R. et al.: Reexamination of testosterone, dihydrotestosterone, estradiol and estrone levels across the menstrual cycle and in postmenopausal women measured by liquid chromatography-tandem mass spectometry. *Steroids* 76:177-82, 2011.

[109] Ziegler R. G., Faupel-Badger J. M., Sue L. Y., Fuhrman B. J. et al.: A new approach to measuring estrogen exposure and metabolism in epidemiologic studies. *J. Steroid Biochem. Mol. Biol.* 121:538-45, 2010.

In: Estrogen Prevention for Breast Cancer
Editor: Zsuzsanna Suba

ISBN: 978-1-62417-378-3

Chapter V

Newly Recognized Player in Breast Cancer Risk: Light Deficiency

Zsuzsanna Suba*

National Institute of Oncology, Department of Surgical and Molecular Pathology, Budapest, Hungary

Abstract

North-America and northern European countries exhibit the highest incidence rate of breast cancer, whereas women in southern regions are relatively protected. Immigrants from low cancer incidence regions to high-incidence areas might exhibit similarly higher or excessive cancer risk as compared with the inhabitants of their adoptive country. Additional cancer risk may be conferred by incongruence between their biological characteristics and foreign environment. Many studies established the racial/ethnic disparities in the risk and nature of female breast cancer in United States between African-American and Caucasian women. Mammary tumors in black women are diagnosed at an earlier age, and are associated with a higher rate of mortality as compared with cancers of white cases. Results of the studies on these ethnic/racial differences in breast cancer incidence suggest that excessive pigmentation of dark skinned women results in a relative light-deficiency. Poor light exposure may explain the deleterious metabolic and hormonal alterations; such as insulin-resistance, deficiencies of estrogen, thyroxin and vitamin-D conferring excessive cancer risk. The more northern the location of an adoptive country, the higher the cancer risk for dark skinned immigrants. Recognition of the deleterious systemic effects of darkness and excessive melatonin synthesis enables cancer protection treatment for people living in light-deficient environment.

* Correspondent author: Prof. Dr. Zsuzsanna Suba, National Institute of Oncology, Surgical and Molecular Tumor Pathology Centre, Address: 1122 Ráth György str. 7-9, Budapest, Hungary. E-mail: subazdr@gmail.com.

Introduction

Cancer epidemiology exhibits great geographic differences suggesting certain causal roles of biological differences in the inhabitants of different lands. Examinations on overall cancer morbidity and mortality data in European countries revealed surprising differences between male and female cases. Countries with the highest male cancer incidence and mortality do not exhibit accumulation in special geographic locations. By contrast, among countries marching at the head in the rank of female overall cancer morbidity and mortality, northern regions are conspicuously highly represented, such as; Denmark, Iceland, Norway and Sweden [1].

This gender-specific excessive risk for overall cancer morbidity and mortality in northern countries raises two possible assumptions. First, there might be noxious factors affecting selectively only the female cases. However, a second possibility is more plausible; common risk factors affect both sexes but women have a peculiar susceptibility to certain cancerogenic agents in northern regions owing to their special hormonal and metabolic features [2].

High incidence of oral cancer among Swedish women as compared with Americans was established in the middle of past century but no causal explanation could be found for this special cancer risk in northern region [3].

Geographic factors seem to have great importance in breast cancer epidemiology as well. There are marked differences among countries in the incidence and mortality rates of breast cancer. Risk for breast cancer is significantly high in the northern regions of America and Europe, whereas in Asia and Africa it is conspicuously low. Incidence and mortality rates of breast cancer are five times higher in the United States than in Japan [4].

Differences in the incidence and mortality rates of breast cancer among countries seem to be both genetic and environmental. Genetic adaptation to a given geographic environment may be a long lasting process and biological selection can have a great role in it. Migration of people shows a typical trend from Southern to Northern, economically highly developed countries. Immigrants move from low cancer incidence regions to high incidence areas, and tend to acquire the cancer incidence rates of their adoptive country, which may mainly be attributed to environmental factors [4]. Conversely, the acquired excessive cancer incidence and mortality rates of dark skinned immigrants might be explained by the incongruence between their biological characteristics and the foreign environment.

African-American women might be regarded as immigrants in the northern part of America as their biologic and genetic characteristics were preserved over centuries. Many studies established the racial/ethnic disparities in the risk and nature of female breast cancer in United States between African-American and Caucasian women [5]. Mammary cancers in black skinned women are diagnosed at an earlier age, their tumors are more aggressive, showing a lower grade of differentiation and the disease exhibits a higher rate of mortality as compared with white cases.

Many investigators tried to explain the excessive risk and the more rapid progression of breast cancer in Afro-American women. Nevertheless, studies suggesting socioeconomic, nutritional, anthropometric, and inherited genetic differences between these ethnic groups were unable to supply confirmatory results [6]. Researchers agree that the clarification of the crucial factors of these ethnic differences should advance understanding breast cancer etiology and finding measures for the primary prevention of breast cancer.

The present study compiles data on differences in breast cancer risk and tumor progression between Afro-American and Caucasian American women based on the results of case-control, prospective and meta-analytic investigations. High acquired cancer risk of dark skinned immigrants in northern countries and Afro-American cases was compared and seemed to exhibit close parallelism.

Differences in Breast Cancer Incidence and Mortality between African-American and White American Women

Strong disparities exist between African-American (AA) and white American (WA) women in the incidence and progression of breast cancer. Among AA women, there is a higher prevalence of breast cancer and more often, the diagnosis is at an earlier age [5]. There are well-known disparities in tumor biology as well. In AA women, mammary tumors are strongly progressive, exhibit lower differentiation and a higher incidence rate of triple negativity as compared with white cases [7]. Tumor recurrence rate, metastatic spread and mortality are all disadvantageous in AA women as compared with either Caucasian or Asian groups in America [5, 8, 9]. Differences in tumor biology between AA and WA women suggested the prevalence of special risk factors for breast cancer in the ethnic group of AA women [6, 8, 9]. In a review of twenty-six research articles, the effect of nutrition, lifestyle and socioeconomic factors were examined in AA and WA cases in correlation with breast cancer incidence. In AA women these parameters were not definitely distinct from those observed in white women [6]. Identification of differentially expressed genes in breast tumors from AA women was compared with those of Caucasian cases. Despite similar pathological characteristics of tumors, molecular profiles exhibited differentially expressed genes in the two ethnic groups of patients, including CRYBB2, PSPHL and SOS1. These genes are involved in cellular growth, differentiation, tumor invasion, metastasis and immune response, thus may contribute to the poor outcome of mammary cancer in AA women [10]. Further studies tried to explain the race and ethnicity disparities in breast cancer cases with the delayed treatment of tumors in black cases [11]. There were differences between black and white women in receiving adjuvant chemotherapy and radiotherapy following tumor removal. Higher risk of mortality in black women as compared to whites was found only in those receiving no chemotherapy [12]. Nevertheless, these treatment differences might be sporadic and don’t explain the disadvantageous morbidity and mortality data of AA women.

Excessive Cancer Risk of African-Americans and Dark Skinned Immigrants in Northern Geographic Regions

Poor light exposure in northern regions means a presumable cancer risk factor for their inhabitants, particularly for women [13]. Predominance of blond, blue eyed, white skinned people in northern regions seems to be a compensatory biological selection as the low level of pigmentation permits more light to pass with higher intensity in case of low exposure to environmental light. However, relatively high cancer morbidity and mortality rates in northern regions reveal that biological compensatory mechanisms are not always sufficient.

Overall cancer morbidity and mortality in Europe exhibited a conspicuously high rate in northern countries among female cases, but not among men [1]. In Northern countries the excessive cancer risk of women as compared with men suggests that the hormonal system of female cases is more sensitive to northern specific risk factors. In Northern Sweden, studies on correlations between obesity and overall cancer risk showed that obese women had a 29.5% excess of risk for developing any malignancy, whereas in obese men there was no significant association between BMI and overall cancer risk [14]. Breast cancer mortality rates were historically lower in the South as compared with the Northeast of United States [15].

Immigrants from southern, low cancer incidence regions to high-incidence northern areas might exhibit similarly increased risk as compared with the inhabitants of their adoptive country, which may be explained by their common environmental factors [4]. By contrast, dark skinned immigrants have markedly higher cancer risk as compared with the natives of northern countries [16, 17]. This excessive risk may be conferred by incongruence between their biological characteristics and the foreign environmental circumstances.

Studies on immigrants may provide valuable insight into the environmental etiology of cancer. In Sweden, the median age of the diagnosis of nasopharyngeal carcinoma (NC) was 63 years old among Swedes and 55 years old among immigrants from South showing a higher risk of the latter group. In black skinned immigrants from North Africa, male cases exhibited highly increased risk (12.4) for NC, whereas women showed extremely high risk (34.7). Among brown skinned Asian Arabic male cases, there was an excessive risk for NC (4.9) and the risk was more than double (10.9) in women [16]. This valuable study reveals that the darker the skin of immigrants the higher their cancer risk in Sweden. Moreover, women exhibit much higher cancer risk as compared with men in each skin color category.

Correlations between ethnicity and age at the time of breast cancer diagnosis were studied on immigrants in Sweden as well. The results showed that in many immigrant groups from South the diagnostic age is earlier (<50) than in natives of Sweden (>50 years) suggesting that true biological factors underlie the differences [17].

Cancer initiation requires a long term exposition to carcinogenic agents. When the patient is debilitated by diverse endocrine defects; such as in cases of black skinned people living in northern regions, the defense mechanisms are weaker and tumor initiation may come earlier. In cases of clinically diagnosed malignancies the imbalance of hormonal mechanisms will disadvantageously affect both the tumor progression and the outcome of the disease.

African-American women might be regarded as southern immigrants in the Northern region of America as their dark pigmentation does not match to the poor light and sunshine of their adoptive country. Excessive breast cancer risk and more rapid tumor progression among African-American women as compared with Caucasians have been thoroughly examined.

Interaction between poor light and excessive defense against light and sunshine by high pigmentation appears to be a strong cancer risk factor both among African-Americans and other dark-skinned immigrants in northern countries. This strong correlation seems to be controversial to the wide-spread concept that excessive light exposure leads to an endocrine disruption and increased breast cancer risk via impaired pineal secretion of melatonin [18].

Traditional Concept Concerning the Oncostatic Capacity of Melatonin Hormone

Pineal hormone melatonin is the mediator of physiological adaptation to external light, and to the day and night rhythms of activity and rest [19]. It seems to be a natural hormone to facilitate sleep as melatonin secretion is physiologically increased in darkness at night being associated with decreased hormonal and metabolic activities. Melatonin administration reduces serum estradiol and thyroxin levels, which suggests that pineal gland is a common neural site to modulate both neuroendocrine-gonadal and neuroendocrine-thyroid axes [20].

Melatonin has an important role in the regulation of reproductive capacity. Melatonin administration may have a contraceptive impact in the female cat by the suppression of gonadotropin releasing hormone (GnRH) production [21]. Conversely, in male cases, hypogonadism mediated by acquired GnRH deficiency is associated with melatonin hypersecretion [22].

Correlations between melatonin and cancer risk are controversial, however the majority of clinical results are supporting its anticancer capacity on hormone dependent tumors [19, 23]. By contrast, carcinogenic activities of melatonin were observed on non-hormone dependent tumors like leukemia. Experimental leukemia exhibited an increased tumor growth by melatonin administration and pinealectomy suppressed leukemic infiltrations in animal experiment [24, 25].

Melatonin administration confers a strong inhibition of estrogen effect by diverse mechanisms and its oncostatic nature has been based on the concept of estrogen induced mammary carcinogenesis [26, 27]. Melatonin is regarded as an oncostatic agent for different kinds of tumors, especially on highly endocrine-responsive breast and endometrial cancers [23, 28]. The most common conclusion is that melatonin reduces the growth of chemically induced mammary tumors in animal experiments. Moreover, melatonin inhibits the proliferation and metastatic behavior of human breast and endometrial cancer cells, in vitro [29-32]. These studies support the oncostatic actions of melatonin on hormone-dependent tumors, which are mainly attributed to its anti-estrogenic actions [26, 27]. Recently, melatonin administration is increasingly suggested for breast cancer therapy because of its presumably advantageous antiestrogenic impact [33].

Correlations between Excessive Melatonin Level, Other Endocrine Functions and Cancer Risk

Associations between Melatonin Excess and Insulin Resistance

Involvement of melatonin in the development of *insulin resistance and diabetes* is poorly understood, whereas there are evidences for its important role in the regulation of glucose uptake [34]. In postmenopausal women, melatonin administration reduced their glucose tolerance and provoked insulin resistance [35]. These observations correctly reflect the decreased insulin sensitivity in correlation with melatonin excess, which means an increased cancer risk particularly for female breast. By contrast, experimental results on rodents suggested antidiabetogenic effects of melatonin treatment [36, 37], improved glucose tolerance and insulin sensitivity in obese diabetic mice [36, 37, 38]. On the other hand, pinealectomy or a removal of melatonin receptors provoked insulin resistance in mice [39, 40].

Circadian insulin secretion is adapted to day/night changes through melatonin-dependent synchronization. In rats and mice, melatonin levels are high during the dark period, which is their active feeding period, while, in humans, melatonin levels are high during the overnight fasting and sleeping period. Melatonin may inversely regulate the day and night changes of glucose uptake and insulin sensitivity in rodents and humans [34]. In a daily active phase (for rodents at night), the melatonin level is low resulting in increased insulin secretion and glucose uptake as well as higher estrogen and thyroxin levels. During inactivity at night (for rodents daytime), a higher melatonin level may be associated with decreased glucose uptake, lower insulin secretion and decreased circulating estrogen and thyroxin levels.

Melatonin has an important impact on diabetes-related metabolc and hormonal disorders [41]. Insulin resistant states, such as metabolic syndrome and type-2 diabetes are in close correlation with carcinogenesis [42-47]. Breast cancer risk is particularly closely associated with these hormonal and metabolic disorders [48-56].

Many studies examined the special inclination for insulin resistance in African-American women as possible explanation for their excessive breast cancer risk. Higher prevalence of metabolic syndrome and type-2 diabetes was observed among African-American women with diagnosed breast cancer as compared with Caucasian cancer cases [52, 57-59]. High plasma insulin concentrations in insulin resistance are associated with alterations in sexual steroid hormone levels as well. There was a significant direct correlation between hyperinsulinism and excessive free testosterone level in young African-American women [58]. Increased prevalence of hyperinsulinemia and the associated relative androgen excess in premenopausal African-American women may have a great role in their excessive breast cancer risk [44, 45, 60].

Obesity, particularly the visceral type is in close correlation with insulin resistance. Obesity and especially the fat deposition on the upper body is more frequent among African-American women and it can partially explain the higher risk and worse prognosis of breast cancer as compared with Caucasian cases [57, 61]. In a study in Los Angeles, associations between BMI defined obesity and breast cancer proved to be significant only among African-American women and was especially significant among postmenopausal cases [62]. These data suggest that obesity and ageing mean higher breast cancer risk for black skinned women as compared with whites in America.

Counteraction between Melatonin Excess and Suppressed Estrogen Signaling Pathways

Estrogen and its signal transduction pathways are the chief regulators of cell proliferation. Embryonic development demonstrates well the omnipotent actions of estrogen [44]. High estrogen levels in pregnant women might ensure explosion-like cell proliferation in the developing embryonic tissues due to the predominance of estrogen receptor alpha signaling pathways. When growth should be stopped, the cessation of mitotic activity results in a dynamic equilibrium of cell number conducted by a concomitant activation of both receptor isoforms. Conversely, by the predominance of estrogen receptor beta activity, a stimulation of apoptotic cell death may induce involution in embryonic structures, which have lost their function. Estrogen deficiency or disorders in estrogen-signaling pathways may elicit a breakdown of the exquisite surveillance of gene regulation and results in cancer initiation [2].

Oncostatic actions of melatonin are predominantly based on the suppression of estrogen-signaling pathways [26, 63, 64]. Melatonin down-regulates the hypothalamic-pituitary reproductive axis by indirect neuroendocrine mechanism resulting in a reduction of circulating gonadal estrogens [20, 26]. Direct effect of melatonin on mammary tumor cells is that it interferes with the activation of nuclear estrogen receptors, thus behaving as a selective estrogen receptor modulator [27, 29-31]. In tumor cell culture, membrane-bound melatonin receptors confer antiestrogenic effects by suppression of estrogen receptor expression [32]. Melatonin may also inhibit the expression and activity of aromatases, the enzymes responsible for the local tissular synthesis of estrogens, thus behaving as a selective enzyme modulator [65].

In hamsters, daily melatonin injections significantly reduced the circulatory serum level of estradiol, rendered female animals acyclic and suppressed their reproductive capacity [20]. Melatonin administration in rats resulted in significant reduction in the number of uterine estrogen receptors, which justifies further counteraction with estrogen effect [66]. On the other hand, estrogen administration exhibited an inhibitory effect on nocturnal melatonin synthesis in peripubertal female rats [67]. Some clinical investigations support the finding that in women suffering of hormone dependent tumors; such as breast or endometrial cancers melatonin levels are depressed [68, 69]. However, these findings should be cautiously evaluated as melatonin secretion is strongly influenced by the age of patients decreasing continuously with aging to about half of the values seen in young people [70].

All experimental data clearly support the counteraction between melatonin and estrogen effects but do not justify that the antiestrogenic impact of melatonin would be protective for hormone related cancers.

Breast cancer risk is increasing with age. In the United States, 75% of women with breast cancer are older than age 50 [4]. Recent clinical and epidemiological results suggest that healthy hormonal equilibrium and fertility are protective for breast cancer in premenopausal women [44]. In estrogen deficient postmenopausal cases, hormone replacement therapy improves the metabolic and hormonal equilibrium and decreases the risk of breast cancer [44, 60].

Hyperinsulinism and defective estrogen signaling are associated with excessive melatonin synthesis in dark skinned American women, which are high cancer risks for female breast. These hormonal alterations might contribute to their increased breast cancer risk [58, 60].

Excessive Melatonin Synthesis and Suppressed Thyroid Function

Melatonin administration induces the suppression of *thyroid function* in animal experiments and in clinical examinations [20]. In melatonin administered hamsters, the serum thyroxin level was reduced to near half that of untreated control animals. Prolonged melatonin treatment in the perimenopausal and early postmenopausal period of women produced a decrease in luteinizing hormone, depressed estradiol level and hypothyroidism [71]. Among patients with hypothyroidism, higher serum melatonin levels, total nocturnal melatonin secretion and urinary melatonin excretion were found as compared with normal control individuals [72].

In a population based study, patients without clinical evidence of thyroid disease were examined to determine whether race or age may influence the serum levels of TSH and free thyroxin (fT4). Mean fT4 value was significantly lower in blacks than in whites, which reveals the wide-spread subclinical hypothyroidism in African-American women [73].

Coincidence of thyroid disorders and breast cancer has long been a subject of debate. Although no convincing evidence exists regarding the causal role for overt thyroid disease in breast cancer, the preponderance of published works favors an association with hypothyroidism [74]. Incidences of thyroid diseases were investigated in patients with breast cancer and age-matched control individuals without breast or thyroid disease. The results indicated an increased prevalence of both autoimmune and non-autoimmune thyroid diseases in breast cancer patients [75]. In a prospective study, hypothyroidism and low serum FT4 values exhibited direct correlation with increased breast cancer risk in postmenopausal women [76]. In animal experiments, hypothyroidism enhanced the invasiveness of breast cancer xenografts and accelerated the development of metastases as well [77]. These associations suggest that low free thyroxin level in black skinned American women may be an additional factor resulting in their excessive breast cancer risk.

Hypothyroidism has a statistically significant relationship with recurrent pregnancy loss in the first trimester [78], suggesting that insufficient thyroid function exhibits correlation with defective estrogen signaling pathway. This association may be a newly revealed link between hypothyroidism and breast cancer risk.

Melatonin Excess Related Vitamin D Deficiency

Melatonin production is enhanced in the darkness at night, whereas vitamin D synthesis is associated with the UV-B spectrum of sunshine. These correlations suggest at least partially opposite actions of these bioactive compounds.

Vitamin D has *beneficial musculoskeletal effects* and crucial extraskeletal ones as well [79]. Vitamin D generates antimicrobial peptide synthesis within epithelial layers of barrier sites, i.e. the respiratory tract, the gastrointestinal tract and skin [80]. Recent prospective studies have shown inverse correlations between serum vitamin D levels and all-cause mortality [81]. In Nordic countries increasing serum vitamin D levels from oral supplementation or ultraviolet-B irradiance mean a marked health benefit [82].

Vitamin D *improves insulin sensitivity*, and its deficiency has been associated with the onset and progression of type-2 diabetes mellitus. Vitamin D3 supplementation might provide a public health measure in preventing or delaying the manifestation of diabetes [83]. Overweight and obese people are insulin resistant and they exhibit lower circulating vitamin D level as compared with cases with normal weight [84]. Vitamin D deficiency is common in children in the United States and is significantly more prevalent in obese children [85].

Vitamin D has important roles in the *reproductive health of women*. Recently, there are literary evidences that vitamin D status influences female fertility and pregnancy outcomes. Low levels of circulatory vitamin D are associated with impaired fertility, polycystic ovarian syndrome, preterm birth and gestational diabetes in women suggesting a defective estrogen signaling pathway in the background. Vitamin D supplementation improves fertility in anovulatory women [86].

Vitamin D was shown to induce *antiproliferative effects* on tumors. In normal and malignant epithelial mammary cells vitamin D has been shown to inhibit pathologic cell proliferation and promote differentiation and apoptosis. Vitamin D deficiency means an increased risk for many cancer types such as; the malignancies of breast, colon, prostate, and pancreas [87, 88]. In cancer patients vitamin D deficiency is associated with a worsening of the prognosis [89]. Vitamin D supplementation was associated with decreased breast cancer incidence, particularly among older postmenopausal women having higher breast cancer risk [90].

Correlations between the *epidemiology of vitamin D supply*, cancer incidence and mortality were studied in the United States [84]. Higher rates of total cancer mortality were observed in regions with less UV-B radiation and among dark-skinned African-American people. A possible role of serum vitamin D3 level emerged in health disparities in black and white cases in United States. Significantly higher ratios of mortality rates for African-Americans to Caucasians were observed for female breast cancer, colorectal cancer, cardiovascular disease and all-cause mortality rate [90]. African-American population exhibits a widespread vitamin D deficiency, which suggests that adequate replacement may be an important public health measure for reduction of race-related disparities in breast cancer incidence [59, 91].

Correlations among Light Exposure, Melatonin Level and Breast Cancer Risk

In *metropolitan inhabitants,* "excessive electric light" exposure at night was supposed to impair the pineal secretion of melatonin [18, 92]. The "endocrine disruption" hypothesis presumed exposure to artificial light at night as a carcinogenic impact by means of defective melatonin synthesis and high circulatory estrogen levels [19, 92]. The hypothesis seemed to be one of the explanations for increased breast cancer risk in highly industrialized regions [93]. However, this concept disregards that electric light at night maybe only a tiny fragment of daylight and sunshine. Moreover, people, staying up the whole night must sleep during the day, resulting in a severe loss of light exposure rather than an excess. This may be the real explanation for their increased cancer risk. Nevertheless, spread of the "western lifestyle" and increased prevalence of insulin resistance and obesity in highly developed countries might be additional high risk for the cancers of breast and other hormone-related sites.

Among *female night shift workers,* an increased breast cancer risk has been observed by several studies [94-97]. This excessive risk was attributed to artificial light exposure at night, defective melatonin secretion and high circulatory estrogen level [98]. However, artificial light at night is negligible in comparison with daylight and female night shift workers sleep during the day. They have a serious deficit of natural light exposure and might suffer of excessive melatonin production with associated hormonal alterations. These systemic disorders really justify their highly increased risk for breast cancer [13]. There is a conspicuous predominance of nurses among night shift workers experiencing breast cancer

[95, 96]. As nurses have the lowest artificial light exposition among women working at night, they are in higher danger of acquiring breast cancer owing to the excessive synthesis of melatonin.

Strongly reduced light exposure and darkness are presumed to be advantageous against cancer via increased melatonin secretion and its antiestrogenic effect. Several studies suggest that *visual impairment and blindness* in women should exhibit lower risk for breast cancer in correlation with their increased melatonin and decreased estrogen levels [19, 99-102]. These results suggest a shocking association that blindness would be advantageous for women to avoid hormone-related cancers. However, the predominance of blond, white skinned and blue eyed persons in northern regions seems to be a compensatory biological selection in case of low exposure to environmental light. This fact justifies that daylight and sunshine are necessary physiological stimuli for human beings and blindness may not be associated with beneficial anticancer capacity. Results suggesting the advantageous anticancer effect of a disability are probably based on preconception and bias.

Taken together, pineal hormone, melatonin seems to be a very important regulator, which harmonizes the diurnal cycles of metabolic and hormonal equilibrium depending on the light exposure and physical activity of living creatures. Darkness and excessive melatonin synthesis results in low estrogen and vitamin D levels, insulin resistance and hypothyroidism, which all seem to be systemic risk factors for cancer.

Conclusion

Literary data on geographic differences in cancer incidence suggest that darkness in northern countries is a gender-related risk for malignancies, particularly among women. Increased cancer morbidity and mortality in northern regions strongly suggest that light and sunshine exposition have important beneficial role in the maintenance of metabolic and endocrine equilibrium. By contrast, literary data suggest an endocrine disruption caused by high estrogen level in light and a beneficial anticancer capacity of long-term darkness. These assumptions are based on the concept that estrogen has carcinogenic capacity, especially on highly hormone responsive organs.

Results of experimental and epidemiological studies exhibit strong correlations between melatonin secretion and the equilibrium of circulatory hormone levels. Health and longevity require a balance and harmony among hormonal signals. Complexity of the endocrine system supplies the high regulation of the proliferative activity of different cell types depending on the nature of temporary intra- and extracellular stimuli.

Literary data on correlations between hormonal disorders and cancer risk are fairly controversial. Overproduction of peptide hormones, such as growth hormone, insulin and insulin-like growth factors, interacting simply with cell membrane receptors, has proven tumor inducing capacity. Another group of hormones, including estrogens, thyroids and vitamin D, has both genomic intranuclear and non-genomic membrane-associated receptor signals, thus they have complex roles in all basic cellular functions. Recent results suggest that defective synthesis of these latter hormones or alterations in their signal transduction pathways may equally disturb metabolic processes, reproduction and the regulation of cell proliferation.

Recognition of the pivotal role of ideal light exposure in human health may supply new insight into the process of carcinogenesis. Deficient light exposure exhibits thorough interplay with systemic cancer risk factors and these correlations illuminate many apparently controversial associations between cancer incidence and hormonal disorders. Moreover, correlations between darkness associated hormonal imbalance and human malignancies supply effective new strategies for primary cancer prevention.

References

[1] Otto Sz. Cancer epidemiology in Hungary and the Béla Johan National Program for the Decade of Health. *Pathol. Oncol. Res.* 9:126-130, 2003.

[2] Suba Z. Common soil of smoking-associated and hormone-related cancers: estrogen deficiency. *Oncol. Rev.* 4:73-87, 2010.

[3] Wynder EL, Bross IJ, Feldman RM. A study of the etiological factors in cancer of the mouth. *Cancer* 10:1300-1323, 1957.

[4] Montag A, Kumar V. The female genital system and breast. Chapter 19. In: Kumar V, Abbas AK, Fausto N, Mitchell RN. Eds. Robbins basic pathology, 8th Ed. Philadelphia, Saunders Elsevier, pp. 711-50, 2007.

[5] Amend K, Hicks D, Ambrosone CB. Breast cancer in African-American women: differences in tumor biology from European-American women. *Cancer Res.* 66:8327-30, 2006.

[6] Chandran U, Hirshfield KM, Bandera EV. The role of anthropometric and nutritional factors on breast cancer risk in African-American women. *Public Health Nutr.* 15:738-48, 2012.

[7] Amirikia KC, Mills P, Bush J, Newman LA. Higher population-based incidence rates of triple-negative breast cancer among young African-American women: Implications for breast cancer screening recommendations. *Cancer* 117:2747-53, 2011.

[8] Stark A, Stapp R, Raghunathan A, Yan X, Kirchner HL, Griggs J et al. Disease-free probability after the first primary ductal carcinoma in situ of the breast: a comparison between African-American and White-American women. *Breast Cancer Res. Treat.* 131:561-70, 2012.

[9] Holmes L Jr, Opara F, Hossain J. A five-year breast cancer-specific survival disadvantage of African American women. *Afr. J. Reprod. Health* 14:195-200, 2010.

[10] Field LA, Love B, Deyarmin B, Hooke JA, Shriver CD, Ellsworth RE. Identification of differentially expressed genes in breast tumors from African-American compared with Caucasian women. *Cancer* 118:1334-44, 2012.

[11] Fedewa SA, Edge SB, Stewart AK, Halpern MT, Marlow NM, Ward EM. Race and ethnicity are associated with delays in breast cancer treatment (2003-2006). *J. Health Care Poor Underserved.* 22:128-41, 2011.

[12] Sail K, Franzini L, Lairson D, Du X. Differences in treatment and survival among African-American and Caucasian women with early stage operable breast cancer. *Ethn. Health* 2011; Nov 9 [Epub ahead of print].

[13] Suba Z. Insulin resistance, hyperinsulinemia and cancer risk. Chapter 2. In: Ed. Suba Z. Estrogen versus Cancer. New York, Nova Science Publishers Inc. pp. 19-40, 2009.

[14] Lukanova A, Björ O, Kaaks R, Lenner P, Lindahl B, Hallmans G et al. Body mass index and cancer: results from the Northern Sweden Health and Disease Cohort. *Int. J. Cancer* 118:458-66, 2006.

[15] Sturgeon SR, Potischman N, Malone KE, Dorgan JF, Daling J, Schairer C et al. Serum levels of sex hormones and breast cancer risk in premenopausal women: a case-control study (USA). *Cancer Causes and Control* 15:45-53, 2004.

[16] Mousavi SM, Sundquist J, Hemminki K. Nasopharyngeal and hypopharyngeal carcinoma risk among immigrants in Sweden. *Int. J. Cancer* 127:2888-92, 2010.

[17] Hemminki K, Mousavi SM, Sundquist J, Brandt A. Does the breast cancer age at diagnosis differ by ethnicity? A study on immigrants to Sweden. *Oncologist* 16:146-54, 2011.

[18] Stevens RG. Electric power use and breast cancer: a hypothesis. *Am. J. Epidemiol.* 125:556-561, 1987.

[19] Rohr UD, Herold J. Melatonin deficiencies in women. *Maturitas* 41:S85-S104, 2002.

[20] Vriend J, Bertalanffy FD, Ralcewicz TA. The effects of melatonin and hypothyroidism on estradiol and gonadotropin levels in female Syrian hamsters. *Biology of Reproduction* 36:719-728, 1987.

[21] Goericke-Pesch S. Reproduction control in cats: new developments in non-surgical methods. *J. Feline Med. Surg*. 12:539-46, 2010.

[22] Luboshitzky R, Shen-Orr Z, Ishai A, Lavie P. Melatonin hypersecretion in male patients with adult-onset idiopathic hypogonadotropic hypogonadism. *Exp. Clin. Endocrinol. Diabetes*. 108:142-5, 2000.

[23] Viswanathan AN, Schernhammer ES. Circulating melatonin and the riskofbreast and endometrial cancer in women. *Cancer Lett.* 281:1-7, 2009.

[24] Bartsch C, Bartsch, Bellmann O, Lippert TH. Depression of serum melatonin in patients with primary breast cancer is not due to an increased peripheral metabolism. *Cancer* 67:1681-4, 1991.

[25] Dreher F, Gabard B, Schwindt DA, Maibach HI. Topical melatonin in combination with vitamin E and C protects skin from ultraviolet-induced erythema. *Br. J. Dermatol.* 139:332-9, 1998.

[26] Cos S. González A. Martínez-Campa C. Mediavilla MD. Alonso-González C. Sánchez-Barceló EJ. Melatonin as a selective estrogen enzyme modulator. *Current Cancer Drug Targets* 8:691-702, 2008.

[27] Cos S, Gonzalez A, Martínez-Campa C, Mediavilla MD, Alonso-González C, Sanchez Barceló EJ. Estrogen signaling pathway: a link between breast cancer and melatonin oncostatic actions. *Cancer Detect. Prev*. 30:118-28, 2006.

[28] Sánchez-Barceló EJ, Cos S, Mediavilla MD, Martinez-Campa C, González A, Alonso-Gozález C. Melatonin-estrogen interactions in breast cancer. *J. Pineal Res*. 38:217-22, 2005.

[29] Hill SM, Frasch T, Xiang S, Yuan L, Duplessis T, Mao L. Molecular mechanisms of melatonin anticancer effects. *Integr. Cancer Ther*. 8:337-46, 2009.

[30] Martínez-Campa C, Alonso-González C, Mediavilla MD, Cos S, González A, Ramos S et al. Melatonin inhibits both ER alpha activation and breast cancer cell proliferation induced by a metallo-estrogen, cadmium. *J. Pineal Res*. 40:291-6, 2006.

[31] Watanabe M, Kobayashi Y, Takahashi N, Kiguchi K, Ishizuka B. Expression of melatonin receptor (MT1) and interaction between melatonin and estrogen in endometrial cancer cell line. *J. Obstet. Gynaecol. Res.* 34:567-73, 2008.
[32] Girgert R, Hanf V, Emons G, Gründker C. Membrane-bound melatonin receptor MT1 down-regulates estrogen responsive genes in breast cancer cells. *J. Pineal Res.* 47:23-31, 2009.
[33] Sanchez-Barcelo EJ, Mediavilla MD, Alonso-Gonzalez C, Rueda N. Breast cancer therapy based on melatonin. *Recent Pat. Endocr. Metab. Immune Drug Discov.* 2012; Febr 20 [Epub ahead of print].
[34] Peschke E, Mühlbauer E. New evidence for a role of melatonin in glucose regulation. *Best Pract. Res. Clin. Endocrinol. Metab.* 24:829-41, 2010.
[35] Cagnacci A, Arangino S, Renzi A, Paoletti AM, Melis GB, Cagnacci P. Influence of melatonin administration on glucose tolerance and insulin sensitivity of postmenopausal women. *Clin. Endocrinol.* 54:339-46, 2001.
[36] Shieh JM, Wu HT, Cheng KC, Cheng JT. Melatonin ameliorates high fat diet-induced diabetes and stimulates glycogen synthesis via a PKCzeta-Akt-GSK3beta pathway in hepatic cells. *J. Pineal Res.* 47:339-44, 2009.
[37] Nishida S, Segawa T, Murai I, Nakagawa S. Long-term melatonin administration reduces hyperinsulinemia and improves the altered fatty-acid compositions in type 2 diabetic rats via the restoration of Delta-5 desaturase activity. *J. Pineal Res.* 32: 26-33, 2002.
[38] Sartori C, Dessen P, Mathieu C, Monney A, Bloch J, Nicod P. Melatonin improves glucose homeostasis and endothelial vascular function in high-fat diet-fed insulin-resistant mice. *Endocrinology* 150:5311-7, 2009.
[39] Contreras-Alcantara S, Baba K, Tosini G. Removal of melatonin receptor type 1 induces insulin resistance in the mouse. *Obesity* (Silver Spring) 18:1861-3, 2010.
[40] Mühlbauer E, Gross E, Labucay K, Wolgast S, Peschke E. Loss of melatonin signaling and its impact on circadian rhythms in mouse organs regulating blood glucose. *Eur. J. Pharmacol.* 606:61-71, 2009.
[41] Espino J, Pariente JA, Rodriguez AB. Role of melatonin on diabetes-related metabolic disorders. *World J. Diabetes* 2:82-91, 2011.
[42] Bloomgarden ZT. Second World Congress on the Insulin Resistance Syndrome: Mediators, pediatric insulin resistance, the polycystic ovary syndrome, and malignancy. *Diabetes Care* 28:1821-1830, 2005.
[43] Suba Z. Insulin resistance and oral cancer risk. *Cancer Res. J.* 3:1-22, 2009.
[44] Suba Z. Interplay between insulin resistance and estrogen deficiency as co-activators in carcinogenesis. *Pathol. Oncol. Res.* 18:123-133, 2012.
[45] Suba Z. Insulin resistance, estrogen deficiency and cancer risk. In: Suba Z Ed. Estrogen versus Cancer. Chapter 7. New York, Nova Science Publishers Inc, pp. 127-146, 2009.
[46] Doyle SL, Donohoe CL, Lysaght J, Reynolds JV. Visceral obesity, metabolic syndrome, insulin resistance and cancer. *Proc. Nutr. Soc.* 71:181-9, 2012.
[47] Grote VA, Becker S, Kaaks R. Diabetes mellitus type 2 – an independent risk factor for cancer? *Exp. Clin. Endocrinol. Diabetes* 118:4-8, 2010.
[48] Rosato V, Bosetti C, Talamini R, Levi F, Montella M, Giacosa A et al. Metabolic syndrome and the risk of breast cancer in postmenopausal women. *Ann. Oncol.* 22: 2687-92, 2011.

[49] Sieri S, Muti P, Claudia A, Berrino F, Pala V, Grioni S et al. Prospective study on the role of glucose metabolism in breast cancer occurrence. *Int. J. Cancer* 130:921-9, 2012.

[50] Abbasi M, Tarafdari A, Esteghamati A, Vejdani K, Nakhiavani M. Insulin resistance and breast carcinogenesis: a cross-sectional study among Iranian women with breast mass. *Metab. Syndr. Relat. Disord.* 8:411-416, 2010.

[51] Gunter MJ, Hoover DR, Yu H, Wassertheil-Smoller S, Rohan TE, Manson JE et al. Insulin, insulin-like growth factor-I, and risk of breast cancer in postmenopausal women. *J. Natl. Cancer Inst.* 101:48-60, 2009.

[52] Colonna SV, Douglas Case L, Lawrence JA. A retrospective review of the metabolic syndrome in women diagnosed with breast cancer and correlation with estrogen receptor. *Breast Cancer Res. Treat.* 131:325-31, 2012.

[53] Vona-Davis L, Howard-McNatt M, Rose DP. Adiposity, type-2 diabetes and the metabolic syndrome in breast cancer. *Obes. Rev.* 8:395-408, 2007.

[54] Arif JM, Al-SaifAM, Al-Karrawi MA, Al-Sagair OA. Causative relationship between diabetes mellitus and breast cancer in various regions of Saudi Arabia: an overview. *Asian Pac. J. Cancer Prev.* 12:589-92, 2011.

[55] Kalla Singh S, Brito C, Tan QW, De León M, De León D. Differential expression and signaling activation of insulin receptor isoforms A and B: A link between breast cancer and diabetes. *Growth Factors* 29:278-89, 2011.

[56] Suba Z. Insulin resistance and oral cancer risk. Chapter 4. In: Watanabe HS. Ed. Horizons in Cancer Research Vol. 43. New York, Nova Science Publishers Inc, pp. 77-97, 2011.

[57] Rose DP, Haffner SM, Baillargeon J. Adiposity, the metabolic syndrome, and breast cancer in African-American and white American women. *Endocr. Rev.* 28:763-77, 2007.

[58] Falkner B, Sherif K, Sumner A, Kushner H. Hyperinsulinism and sex hormones in young adult African Americans. *Metabolism* 48:107-12, 1999.

[59] Harris SS. Does vitamin D deficiency contribute to increased rates of cardiovascular disease and type 2 diabetes in African Americans? *Am. J. Clin. Nutr.* 93:1175S-78S, 2011.

[60] Suba Z, Kásler M. Interactions of insulin and estrogen in the regulation of cell proliferation and carcinogenesis. *Orv. Hetil.* (in Hungarian) 153:47-58, 2012.

[61] Conroy SM, Maskarinec G, Wilkens LR, White KK, Henderson BE, Kolonel LN. Obesity and breast cancer survival in ethnically diverse postmenopausal women: the Multiethnic Cohort Study. *Breast Cancer Res. Treat.* 129:565-74, 2011.

[62] *Sarkissyan M, Wu Y, Vadgama* JV. Obesity is associated with breast cancer in African-American women but not Hispanic women in South Los Angeles. *Cancer* 117:3814-23, 2011.

[63] Sandyk R, Anastasiadis PG, Anninos PA, Tsagas N. Is the pineal gland involved in the pathogenesis of endometrial carcinoma. *Int. J. Neurosci.* 62:89-96, 1992.

[64] Grant SG, Melan MA, Latimer JJ, Witt-Enderby PA. Melatonin and breast cancer: cellular mechanisms, clinical studies and future perspectives. *Expert Rev. Mol.* 11:e5, 2009.

[65] Gonzalez A, Cos S, Martinez-Campa C, Alonso-Gonzalez C, Sanchez-Mateos S, Mediavilla MD. Selective estrogen enzyme modulator actions of melatonin in human breast cancer cells. *J. Pineal Res.* 45:86-92, 2008.

[66] Abd-Allah AR, El-Sayed el SM, Abdel-Wahab MH, Hamada FM. Effect of melatonin on estrogen and progesterone receptors in relation to uterine contraction in rats. *Pharmacol. Res.* 47:349-354, 2003.

[67] Hayashi K, Okatani Y. Mechanisms underlying the effects of estrogen on nocturnal melatonin synthesis in peripubertal female rats: relation to norepinephrine and adenylatecyclase. *J. Pineal Res.* 26:178:83, 1999.

[68] Grin W, Grünberger W. A significant correlation between melatonin deficiency and endometrium cancer. *Gynecol. Obstet. Invest.* 45:62-5, 1998.

[69] Bartsch C, Bartsch H, Blask DE, Cardinali DP, Hrushewsky WJM, Mecke D. The pineal gland and cancer. Springer: Berlin 2001.

[70] Ohashi Y, Okamoto N, Uchida K, Iyo M, Mori N, Morita Y. Differential pattern of the circadian rhythm of serum melatonin in young and elderly healthy subjects. *Biol. Signals* 6:301-6, 1997.

[71] Bellipani G, Bianchi P, Pierpaoli W, Bulian D, Ilyia E. Effects of melatonin in perimenopausal women and menopausal women: a randomized and placebo controlled study. *Exp. Gerontol.* 36:297-310, 2001.

[72] Röjdmark S, Berg A, Rössner S, Wetterberg L. Nocturnal melatonin secretion in thyroid disease and in obesity. *Clin. Endocrinol.* 35:61-65, 1991.

[73] Boucai L, Surks MI. Reference limits of serum TSH and free T4 are significantly influenced by race and age in an urban outpatient medical practice. *Clin. Endocrinol.* (Oxf) 70:788-93, 2009.

[74] Smyth PP. The thyroid and breast cancer: a significant association? *Ann. Med.* 29:189-91, 1997.

[75] Turken O, Narin Y, Demirbas S, Onde ME, Sayan O, Kandemir EG et al. Breast cancer in association with thyroid disorders. *Breast Cancer Res.* 5:R110-113, 2003.

[76] Kuijpens JL, Nyklictek I, Louwman MW, Weetman TA, Pop VJ, Coebergh JW. Hypothyroidism might be related to breast cancer in post-menopausal women. *Thyroid* 15:1253-9, 2005.

[77] Martinez-Inglesias O, Garcia-Silva S, Regadera J, Aranda A. Hypothyroidism enhances tumor invasiveness and metastasis development. *PLoS One* 4:e6428, 2009.

[78] Rao VR, Lakshmi A, Sadhnani MD. Prevalence of hypothyroidism in recurrent pregnancy loss in first trimester. *Indian J. Med. Sci.* 62:357-61, 2008.

[79] Dobnig H. A review of the health consequences of the vitamin D deficiency pandemic. *J. Neurol. Sci.* 311:15-18, 2011.

[80] White JH. Vitamin D as an inducer of cathelicidin antimicrobial peptide expression: past, present and future. *J. Steroid Biochem. Mol. Biol.* 121:234-8, 2010.

[81] Melamed ML, Michos ED, Post W, Astor B. 25-Hydroxyvitamin D levels and the risk of mortality in the general population. *Arch. Intern. Med.* 168:1629-37, 2008.

[82] Grant WB, Juzeninene A, Moan JE. Review article: Health benefit of increased serum 25 (OH)D levels from oral intake and ultraviolet-B irradiance in the Nordic countries. *Scand. J. Public Health* 39:70-78, 2011.

[83] Nazarian S, St Peter JV, Boston RC, Jones SA, Mariash CN. Vitamin D3 supplementation improves insulin sensitivity in subjects with impaired fasting glucose. *Transl. Res.* 158:276-81, 2011.

[84] Giovanucci E. The epidemiology of vitamin D and cancer incidence and mortality: a review (United States). *Cancer Causes Control* 16:83-95, 2005.

[85] Olson ML, Maalouf NM, Oden JD, White PC, Hutchinson MR. Vitamin D deficiency in obese children and its relationship to glucose homeostasis. *J. Clin. Endocrinol. Metab*. 97:279-85, 2012.

[86] Grundmann M, von Versen-Höynck F. Vitamin D – roles in women's reproductive health? *Reprod. Biol. Endocrinol*. 9:146-55, 2011.

[87] Mitchell D. The relationship between vitamin D and cancer. *Clin. J. Oncol. Nurs* 15: 557-60, 2011.

[88] Pilz S, Tomaschitz A, Obermayer-Pietsch B, Dobnig H, Pieber TR. Epidemiology of vitamin D insufficiency and cancer mortality. *Anicancer Res*. 29:3699-704, 2009.

[89] Arends J. Vitamin D in oncology. *Forsch Komplementmed* 18:176-84, 2011.

[90] Crew KD, Gammon MD, Steck SE, Hershman DL, Cremers S, Dworakowski E et al. Association between plasma 25-hydroxyvitamin D and breast cancer risk. *Cancer Prev. Res*. (Phila) 2:598-604, 2009.

[91] Grant WB, Peiris AN. Possible role of serum 25-hydroxyvitamin D in black-white health disparities in the United States. *J. Am. Med. Dir. Assoc*. 11:617-28, 2010.

[92] Stevens RG. Working against our endogenous circadian clock: Breast cancer and electric lighting in the modern world. *Mutat. Res*. 680:106-108, 2009.

[93] Cohen M, Lippman M, Chabner B. Role of pineal gland in aetiology and treatment of breast cancer. *Lancet* 2:814-6, 1978.

[94] Bonde JP, Hansen J, Kolstad HA, Mikkelsen S, Olsen JH, Blask DE et al. Work at night and breast cancer – report on evidence-based options for preventive actions. *Scand. J. Work Environ. Health* 2012; Feb 20 [Epub ahead of print].

[95] Langley AR, Graham CH, Grundy AL, Tranmer JE, Richardson H, Aronson KJ. A cross sectional study of breast cancer biomarkers among shift working nurses. *BMJ* Open Jan 21;2:e000532, 2012.

[96] Grundy A, Tranmer J, Richardson H, Graham CH, Aronson KL. The influence of light and night exposure on melatonin levels among Canadian rotating shift nurses. *Cancer Epidemiol. Biomarkers Prev*. 20:2404-12, 2011.

[97] Brudnowska J, Peplonska B. Night shift work and cancer risk: a literature review (Polish). *Med. Pr*. 62:323-38, 2011.

[98] Blask DE, Brainard GC, Dauchy RT, Hanifin JP, Davidson LK, Krause JA et al. Melatonin-depleted blood from premenopausal women exposed to light at night stimulates growth of human breast cancer xenografts in nude rats. *Cancer Res*. 65: 11174-11184, 2005.

[99] Kliukiene J, Tynes T, Andersen A. A risk of breast cancer among women with visual impairment. *Br. J. Cancer* 84:397-9, 2001.

[100] Hahn RA. Profound bilateral blindness and incidence of breast cancer. *Epidemiology* 2:208-10, 1991.

[101] Feychting M, Osterlund B, Ahlbom A. Reduced cancer incidence among the blind. *Epidemiology* 9:490-4, 1998.

[102] Verkasalo PK, Pukkala E, Stevens RG, Ojamo M, Rudanko SL. Inverse association between breast cancer incidence and degree of visual impairment in Finland. *Br. J. Cance*r 80:1459-60, 1999.

In: Estrogen Prevention for Breast Cancer
Editor: Zsuzsanna Suba

ISBN: 978-1-62417-378-3

Chapter VI

Estrogen Prevention of Breast Cancer: A Critical Review

Joseph Ragaz* and Shayan Shakeraneh#
University of British Columbia, B. C., Canada

Abstract

This chapter articulates an evolving paradigm: Estrogen, historically and presently considered the main human breast carcinogen confers paradoxically a statistically significant reduction of the incidence of invasive breast cancer rates. [1] Furthermore, the most recent update of the Women's Health Initiative [WHI] trial of estrogen alone versus placebo in women with hysterectomy confirms also a significant reduction of breast cancer mortality. [2]

Thus, the use of Hormone Replacement Therapy [HRT] based on estrogen alone deserves serious merits for breast cancer chemoprevention. [3] Furthermore, if started at the age 50-60 to manage menopausal symptoms, estrogen-based HRT will result in a significant reduction of myocardial infarction and coronary heart disease, [1] leading thus to a significant reduction of all-cause mortality. [2] These essential health outcome gains are all in addition to the well documented quality of life improvement due to amelioration of menopausal symptoms.

Supportive evidence for the breast cancer rate reduction due to Estrogen comes from emerging basic research studies: estrogen has recently shown to exhibit an inverse link with carcinogenic co-factors such as insulin growth factor one [IGF-1], [4] as well as a beneficial role on human stem cells. [5]

And importantly, there is rising recognition of its role in apoptosis, [6] particularly after prior estrogen deprivation. [7,8]

Despite the strong levels of evidence for cumulative benefits to women entering menopause, physicians and public at large are hardly aware of these gains.

* Corresponding author: Dr.Joseph Ragaz, School of Population and Public Health, University of British Columbia [B. C.], 2206 East Mall Vancouver, B.C., V6T 1Z3, Canada; Tel.:604 5692446; e-mail: joseph.ragaz@ubc.ca;
# Second author E-mail: *shayans@interchange.ubc.ca.*

HRT whether the combination of estrogen+provera or estrogen alone, is continuously surrounded by a strong guideline negativism, with the century old concept of estrogen as the main breast carcinogen and HRT harm exceeding benefit basically unaltered.

This review does not discuss in depth the data of HRT based on estrogen plus progestin combination - the WHI first randomized trial; nor does it review the HRT-estrogen alone outcomes based on the observational non-randomized studies. The structure and outcomes of these other studies differ from the WHI estrogen-alone trial, with the complexities of adjusting for the multitude of confounding factors, challenges of inter-trial comparisons, and in particular, biases related to non-randomized study designs clearly exceeding the scope of this review.

Rather, this chapter offers a more detailed emerging evidence for estrogen impact in women entering menopause as identified from the update of the only randomized trial of estrogen versus placebo in existence. [1,2].

And specifically, as the book title indicates, the chapter is focusing on the newly emerging issue of estrogen role in the prevention of breast cancer - one of the most important newly evolving paradigms in science.

Background: Randomized HRT WHI Trials

The Women's Health Initiative [WHI] HRT trials were planned in the early parts of the 1990's because of rising concerns that past HRT observational and case-controlled studies were based on small patient sample size or on study results with pre-selected participants who could be in a better state of health than women who were not eligible for HRT. Thus, the objectives of the WHI HRT studies were to determine, from large randomized trials, the individual HRT-related outcomes, in order to influence the clinical practice whereby HRT was increasingly since the 1980's prescribed not only for the palliation of postmenopausal symptoms, but also for reduction of heart disease, cardiac mortality, and in general, to slow down the aging-related chronic degenerative conditions and improving all-cause mortality reduction. [9-11] Paradoxically, published were also preliminary data showing that despite the increased breast cancer incidence rates, there could also be a reduction of breast cancer mortality. [11]

The WHI project is perhaps the most extensive population research, based on randomized controlled studies of healthy female population, to evaluate the health benefits and risks among 68,132 postmenopausal women in the age range 50–79 at randomization. Enrollment into the WHI began in 1993 and concluded in 1998 with the first two of the four trials focusing on the HRT. The four WHI randomized controlled clinical trials included:

1. *TRIAL ONE* involved Hormone Replacement Therapy (HRT), testing in healthy women and with intact uterus the impact of estrogen – the Conjugated Equine Estrogen (CEE, Premarin, 0.625 mg/day) plus progestin (medroxyprogesterone acetate 2.5 mg/day) versus a placebo. The primary objective was to determine the HRT impact on coronary heart disease prevention, with breast cancer as an anticipated adverse effect. Additional HRT related conditions constituted secondary objectives of this trial. Overall, 16, 608 women were randomized to this trial.

2. *TRIAL TWO* was designed for women without uterus and randomized to Estrogen alone with CEE versus placebo, with the same objectives as TRIAL ONE. Altogether, 10,739 women were recruited to this trial. Our review is focused on the outcomes of this particular trial.
3. *TRIAL THREE* tested low-fat against conventional diet for breast and colorectal cancer prevention, with 48,835 women randomized.
4. *TRIAL FOUR* tested the impact of calcium and vitamin D supplementation. Hip fractures were the designated primary outcome, with other fractures and colorectal cancer as secondary outcomes. In total, 36,282 women were randomized to this trial.

The WHI program also includes an observational study (ObSt) that comprised additional 93,676 postmenopausal women recruited from the same population base as the randomized trials. The ObSt is intended to provide additional knowledge about risk factors for a range of diseases, including cancer, cardiovascular disease, and fractures. It has an emphasis on biological markers of disease risk and on risk-factor changes as risk modifiers.

WHI HRT Results - Trial 1, Estrogen + Provera vs Placebo

The July 17, 2002 JAMA article reported the results of the first HRT trial – the estrogen plus progestin (E2+Prog) versus placebo. [12] The primary outcome measures were events related to incident cases of:

1. Coronary Heart Disease – CHD (EVENT 1).
2. Invasive Breast Cancer (EVENT 2).

This trial was terminated unexpectedly on the weight of interim data, on the advice of the independent Data and Safety Monitoring Board, after a mean 5.2 years of follow-up, because of an increased risk of breast cancer and an overall assessment of "harms exceeding benefits" for chronic disease prevention.

Specifically, as increased harm, reported were a 26% increase in breast cancer incidence; 29% increase of CHD; 41% increase in risk of stroke and a doubling of the rates of thromboembolism.

None of these hazards, with the exception of thromboembolism, were increased with statistical significance.

As reduction of harm, there was a significant 25% reduction of skeletal fracture rates; a 37% reduction of colorectal cancer; a 17% reduction of endometrial cancer; and a 2% reduction of deaths from any cause.

However, despite these benefits, the Global Index, an interactive summary of harms and benefits, was increased (HR=1.15, 95% C.I.=0.95-1.39).

Thus, authors concluded that for an average 5.2 years follow-up time:

1. Overall health risks of combined estrogen plus progestin exceeded benefits among healthy postmenopausal US women.
2. All-cause mortality was not different between the two groups.

3. The risk-benefit profile is not consistent with the requirements for an intervention for primary prevention of chronic diseases such as CHD.

WHI HRT RESULTS – TRIAL 2, ESTROGEN Alone vs PLACEBO in Women after Hysterectomy

Despite the early termination of the first WHI estrogen plus progestin trial in 2002, the second WHI estrogen-alone trial was continued. As in the first trial, of all participants, only less than one third (30.8%) in the second trial were <60 years of age; and over 47% were past or current HRT users before enrollment. Approximately 40% of all participants had oophorectomy with hysterectomy (39.5% vs 42% in arm of CEE vs placebo, respectively). Forty eight percent of women in the trial had been treated for hypertension and 15% had therapy for elevated cholesterol. Overall, 86% of all patients had no first degree relative with breast cancer; and 74.5% had no benign breast disease in the past.

At the time of the first analysis, in 2004, taking all participants, the estimated hazard ratios (with Adjusted 95% Confidence Intervals) for estrogen alone vs placebo showed a 9% reduction of CHD; a 33% (non-significant) increase in thromboembolism; a 39% increase in strokes; and an 8% increase in colorectal cancer.

However, reduced were the rates of breast cancer, by 23% and of overall skeletal fractures primarily of hip fractures, by a significant 39% %. Total death rate was increased non-significantly, by 4%; and so was the Global Index, by 1%. For the crude outcomes, there was an absolute excess risk of 12 additional strokes per 10,000 person-years and an absolute risk reduction of 6 fewer hip fractures per 10,000 person-years. The estimated risk for all monitored events in the Global Index was a non-significant excess of 2 events per 10,000 person-years.

On account of these results, the second WHI trial on CEE alone vs placebo concluded that the use of CEE, in women after hysterectomy, after follow-up of 6.8 years:

a. Increases the risk of strokes.
b. Decreases the risk of hip fracture.
c. Does not affect the CHD incidence.
d. May lead to a possible reduction in breast cancer risk requiring further investigation.
e. The sum of combined events was equivalent in the CEE and placebo groups, indicating no overall benefit and no hazards.

In the final conclusion, the authors stated that estrogen alone with CEE "should not be recommended for chronic disease prevention in postmenopausal women." [13]

As a result of these data and recommendations, after reviewing data through November 30, 2003, the National Institutes of Health (NIH) decided in February 2004 to end the intervention phase of the second WHI HRT trial early, with results published in the April 14, 2004 issue of the Journal of American Medical Association. [13].

Table 1. WHI trial 1 - HRT with CEE plus MPA (medroxyprogeterone) versus Placebo Total Mortality, Coronary Heart Disease and Strokes, According to Years from the Menopause. Modified, from Rossouw *et al.* [16]

Total Mortality

Years since Menopause	HRT%	Placebo%	RR	95% CI
<10	0.24	0.31	0.76	0.53-1.09
10-19	0.53	0.55	0.98	0.78-1.24
>20	1.05	0.93	1.14	0.96-1.36

CHD

Years since Menopause	HRT%	Placebo%	RR	95% CI
<10	18	0.24	0.76	0.50-1.16
10-19	0.43	0.39	1.10	0.84-1.45
>20	0.78	0.62	1.28	1.03- 1.58

Strokes – Incidence

Years since menopause	HRT%	Placebo%	RR	95% CI
<10	0.19	0.11	1.77	1.05- 2.98
10-19	0.38	0.30	1.23	0.92- 1.66
>20	0.57	.044	1.26	0.98- 1.66

Critique of the WHI HRT Trial Reporting

Overall Outcomes - Age 50-59 versus Older Age Groups

The sudden move to halt prescribing HRT was soon followed by reports of substantial breast cancer incidence reduction in the US population after 2002. [14] However, several publications raised the issue of prematurely stopping the HRT trials, and suggested caution in the WHI HRT trials' interpretation. [15] But the adverse HRT reports continued, despite the fact that data from the first WHI HRT trial showing for younger women age 50 – 60, the age where HRT is actually indicated to manage menopause, the hazards of total mortality were substantially reduced (Table 1), with a statistically significant 30% reduction of all-cause mortality (HR = 0.70; 95% C.I.= 0.51-0.96). [16] Similarly, CHD and strokes, the principal two events responsible for halting the first HRT trial, were not adversely affected among women age 50-59.

And the second WHI trial? Already at the time of the first 2004 – 2006 reports, [13,17] the analysis restricted to the age group 50 to 69 showed a 44% reduction of CHD events approaching statistical significance (HR=0.56, 0.30-1.03). [13] As with the first WHI trial, strokes were also not increased among young women age 50-69 (HR=1.08, 95% C.I.=0.57-2.04). Bone fractures, among all participants (except the women <age 60 with very few events) were reduced consistently and with statistical significance, with trends for more protection among younger women (HR=0.33, for the ages 60-69 versus HR= 0.62, for ages 70-79), accounting for 38-67% reduction of bone fractures – an important contributory factor

towards all-cause mortality in women. And indeed, already in 2004, total death rates were reduced by 27% among young women age 50-69. [13]

Estrogen and the Rates of Invasive Breast Cancer

The unexpected yet potentially most important aspect of the WHI's second HRT trial involved invasive breast cancer analyses. Taking all trial participants, the hazard rates of invasive breast cancer were reduced by 23% - a reduction approaching statistical significance already in 2004 (HR=0.77, 95% C.I.= 0.59-1.01). However, because of the reports by the WHI describing these potential gains as "absence of harm" rather than potential major benefits, the medical establishment at large and the lay public remained unaware.

And the situation persists basically until today, despite the fact that the new 2011 – 2012 WHI HRT updates of trial 2 confirms statistical significance to the breast cancer rate reduction by estrogen, and thus a potential for a major estrogen impact in breast cancer prevention, in addition to the dents in mortality and for quality of life benefits to women entering menopause.

But before the new update review, let's identify the role of Estrogen in the established breast cancer, in the setting of stage IV advanced disease, and also provide some new evidence of estrogen benefit identified from the basic research.

Estrogen Benefit in Human Breast Cancer – Clinical Stage IV Breast Cancer

Using estrogen alone to treat advanced breast cancer is not new: high-dose synthetic estrogen diethylstilbestrol (DES) was a mainstay in hormonal treatment of metastatic breast cancer since the late 1940's, and became the main single hormonal agent to treat stage IV breast cancer until the development in mid-1970's of tamoxifen. [6,18,19] DES in metastatic breast cancer produced reproducible 20-30% response rates [6,18,19] with limiting factors thrombo-embolic episodes and pulmonary emboli, as well as nausea, and endometrial stimulation with menorrhagia. Its use was abandoned in the late 1970's when randomized and non-randomized trials confirmed comparable or superior rates of tamoxifen, an agent with considerably lower rates of thromboembolism and nausea. [20]

The initial explanation of mechanism of estrogen action was articulated from an *in-vitro* study by Lippmann *et al.* showing in MCF-7 *in-vitro* cell lines an initial stimulation by low-dose estrogen; however as the dose of estrogen was escalated, the stimulation rate decreased, and high estrogen dose was tumor suppressive. [21]

This observation was confirmed by a clinical 1977 study of Carter *et al.* [22] of 523 postmenopausal patients with stage IV breast cancer. Patients were randomized to four different dosages of diethylstilbestrol: 1.5, 15, 150, or 1,500 mg/day, with results showing highest response [21%] for the highest dose; and lowest response rate [10%] for the lowest dose. [22]

Contrary conclusion about estrogen dose-response was reached, however, by more recent randomized trial of Ellis *et al.* who randomized 6 mg vs 30 mg of oral estradiol used daily. [23] All 66 randomized patients had metastatic breast cancer and were treated with an aromatase inhibitor before the study start. Results showed the adverse event rate (grade 3) in the 30-mg group to be significantly higher (11/32 [34%]; than in the 6-mg group (4/34 [18%]; P=.03). However, clinical benefit rates were equivalent in the 6-mg group, with 29% response rate versus 28% in the 30-mg group, confirming that clinically acceptable lower estrogen dose with minimal side effects is actually equivalent to the higher dose, with substantially more toxicity.

A final evidence for estrogen benefit in established human cancer comes from an update [24] of a study initiated already in the 1970's at Mayo Clinic of 143 stage IV breast cancer patients randomized between estrogen (DES) or tamoxifen (TAM) as single hormonal treatments. [25] While the initial 1981 report of 5 year follow-up [with 31% of the trial patients dead] confirmed equivalence, and higher toxicity of stilboestrol [25], the long-term update with 15 year follow-up [>95% of study patients dead] showed survival outcome benefit of estrogen over tamoxifen. Adjusting for other contributing factors, the long-term survival of women on estrogen was significantly longer, at 3.0 years vs a median survival of 2.4 years for women on tamoxifen, with prorated estimates of 44% increased rate of deaths in the tamoxifen arm over stilboestrol [HR=1.44, 95% C.I.=1.02-2.03]. This important update confirms the long-term follow-up superiority of estrogen over tamoxifen in reducing breast cancer related mortality over what has been considered a first line breast cancer hormonal agent until recently.

Estrogen Benefit in Breast Cancer: Basic Research Data and Mechanism of Action

The issue regarding estrogen and breast carcinogenesis therefore at present is not any more *if* estrogen is effective, but the mechanism of its action. Initially, as per Lippman *et al.* [21], estrogen benefit was considered a function of dose: low-dose estrogen stimulates; high dose would suppress. This potentially attractive concept has been now modified by the above randomized trial of Ellis *et al.* [23] showing no dose-response effect of estrogen, with 6 mg showing equivalence with the high dose of 30 mg.

One of the most influential recent suggestions explaining conditions for estrogen benefit comes from the Santen group. [7,8] Santen *et al.* and Song *et al.* proposed the estrogen benefit to be restricted to breast cancer cells with prior estrogen deprivation: in estrogen deprived cells, in the *in-vitro* setting, estrogen leads to cancer deaths and thus to prevention. Estrogen deprivation therapy in the clinical setting such as after aromatase inhibitors - a classical anti-estrogenic approach - has been thus hypothesized to paradoxically sensitize hormone-receptor-positive breast cancer tumor cells to low-dose estradiol therapy. [7]

Jordan *et al.* published on estrogen mechanism of action identifying enhanced apoptosis in breast cancer cells after estrogen therapy under certain conditions. [26] While the mechanisms by which estrogen induces apoptosis are still not completely known, recent evidence demonstrated the involvement of different apoptotic signaling including the NF-κB (nuclear factor-kappa-B)-mediated survival pathway as well as the PI3K (phosphoinositide 3-

kinase)/Akt signaling pathways, with particular implications for beneficial impact with low-dose estrogen.

Lastly, the group of Vivanco *et al.* [5] showed additional scale of importance: estrogen activity leads to the suppression of stem cells; and Suba reviewed a potentially very important link between estrogen deprivation and activation of insulin axis as a model for human carcinogenesis, [27] not only for breast cancer, but also lung, oral and perhaps a scale of other epithelial malignancies. [28]

Estrogen in Prevention of Breast Cancer? The Final 2000 – 2012 Reports

Until 2009, no real attempt was made to highlight the significance of the emerging breast cancer rate reduction by estrogen alone seen in the WHI HRT trial two, complementing the response rates in stage IV breast cancer by stilboestrol and matched by estrogen data on breast cancer cells *in vitro*. Overall emphasis remained on "absence of harm" rather than on "evidence for benefit." In 2009 – 2010, Ragaz *et al.* reviewed all the WHI HRT trials as published between 2004 – 2006, [3,29] emphasizing a qualitatively different set of conclusion: estrogen actually confers a major benefit: observed is, overall, a breast cancer risk reduction of at least 20%. However, the 79.6% trial participants without past history of benign disease – i.e. the majority of trial participants, had a significant 43% reduction of invasive breast cancer by HRT (HR=0.57, 95% C.I.=0.41-0.78) (Table 2a). Similarly, women without history of first degree relative of breast cancer (86% of the trial population), had a statistically significant 32% reduction of invasive breast cancer with estrogen alone (HR=0.68, 95% C.I.=0.50-0.92) (Table 2b).

As a result, the British Columbia team articulated a paradigm changing proposal: *Exogenous* estrogen is breast cancer protective while *endogenous* estrogen remains carcinogenic, with *exogenous* estrogen deserving merits for chemoprevention. [3] Despite the strengths of these data, and some publicity by scientific and lay media,* no change in guidelines, however, followed.

WHI reports 2011 – 2012. Two definitive WHI HRT updates of the second Estrogen-alone vs. placebo trial were published in 2011 [1] and 2012. [2]

First, LaCroix *et al.* reported in JAMA 2011 results after a median follow-up of 11.8 years. This time, among women age 50-59, the true HRT candidates as they enter menopause, a significant 46% reduction of myocardial infarction was shown due to estrogen [HR=0.54, 95% C.I.= 0.34-0.86], with a 29% reduction of deep vein thrombosis [HR=0.71, 95% C.I.=0.40-1.26], no increase in stroke [HR=1.09], and to a 27% reduction of overall mortality reaching statistical significance [HR = 0.73; 95% C.I.= 0.53-1.00]. And the breast cancer rate reduction due to estrogen – perhaps the most contentious issues of the whole WHI program - continued, now with a significant 23% reduction of hazards [HR=0.77, 95% CI = 0.62-0.95].

---

*http://www.aacr.org/home/public--media/aacr-in-the-news.aspx?d=2218.
http://www.nytimes.com/2010/12/14/health/research/14hormone.html?_r=3&ref=health.

Table 2. Rates of Invasive Breast Cancer, WHI 2nd Trial [CEE vs Placebo] Impact of Prior Breast Cancer Risk. Report by Ragaz *et al.* [3], Modified from Stefanick *et al.*, 2006 [17]

Table 2a. Prior Risk for Breast Cancer Determined by History of Benign Breast Disease

Past Benign Breast Disease	CEE	Placebo	HR	95% CI
No	0.23%	0.39%	0.57	0.41 – 0.78
Yes, 1 Biopsy	0.45%	0.29%	1.60	0.82 – 3.14
Yes, >1 Biopsy	0.41%	0.19%	2.54	0.73 – 8.86

Table 2b. Prior Risk for Breast Cancer Determined by First Degree Relative with Breast Cancer

First Degree Relative with Breast Cancer	CEE	Placebo	HR	95% CI
None	0.23%	0.34%	0.68	0.50 – 0.92
>1	0.41%	0.19%	2.54	0.73 – 8.86

These benefits, however, are again not highlighted, they are summarized as "...among younger women, *no new safety concerns* emerged and *some risk reductions* became apparent during the post-intervention period" and that "mechanisms underlying the reduced risks of breast cancer in all women, and coronary events in younger but not older women, warrant further study." [1]

The last update of the same estrogen-alone trial focusing more on breast cancer outcomes was published in March 2012. [2] In this, taking all participants as randomized, the use of estrogen was associated for the first time with a statistically significant *breast cancer mortality reduction* [HR=0.37, 95% C.I. =0.13-0.91], and, with *all-cause mortality reduction* (a 38% reduction of risk of deaths from any cause, HR=0.62, 95% C.I., 0.39-0.97; p=0.04). As in the prior British Columbia team's 2010 presentation, [3] breast cancer risk reduction was highly significant among the 80% of women without benign breast disease [HR=0.61, 95% C.I.=0.47-0.79], and among women without a first degree family history of breast cancer [HR=0.68, 95% C.I. = 0.53-0.88].

Conclusion

This review shows, that taking all the emerging clinical data, there is a documented statistically significant benefit of estrogen on the rates of invasive breast cancer in healthy women after hysterectomy, complementing the prior evidence for reduction of breast cancer burden in established stage IV breast cancer. These data imply the potential of *exogenous* estrogen for actual prevention of breast carcinogenesis, while they do not challenge the prior data from multiple randomized studies confirming with evidence level 1 association of *endogenous* estrogen as the pivotal breast carcinogen [30,31].

At this time multiple questions remain unanswered in regards to basic science of estrogen mechanisms for these activities and or selection for optimum hormonal regimens to manage menopause. However, this review shows, that the prior 2010 proposal of a *dual effect of estrogen* regarding human breast cancer, [3] is not a hypothesis anymore, but rather a clinically validated observation based on strong levels of evidence identified from randomized trials.

These data indicate that HRT guidelines may need to embrace *exogenous* estrogen as a potentially pivotal agent for breast cancer prevention, associated with multiple health outcome benefits for women entering menopause including all-cause mortality reduction. The medical establishment and lay public need to be aware of these data, with those responsible for execution of public health policies facing an obligation of disseminating these conclusions effectively to women entering menopause.

References

[1] LaCroix A. Z., Chlebowski R. T., Manson J. E., et al. Health outcomes after stopping conjugated equine estrogens among postmenopaUSl women with prior hysterectomy: a randomized controlled trial. *Jama* 2011;305:1305-14.

[2] Anderson G. L., Chlebowski R. T., Aragaki A. K., et al. Conjugated equine oestrogen and breast cancer incidence and mortality in postmenopaUSl women with hysterectomy: extended follow-up of the Women's Health Initiative randomised placebo-controlled trial. *Lancet Oncol.* 2012;13:476-86.

[3] Ragaz J., Wilson K., Muraca G., Budlovsky J., Froehlich J. Dual estrogen effects on breast cancer: endogenous estrogen stimulates, exogenous estrogen protects. Further investigation of estrogen chemoprevention is warranted. *Cancer Res.* 2010;70.

[4] Suba Z. Interplay Between Insulin Resistance and Estrogen Deficiency as co-Activators in Carcinogenesis. *Pathol. Oncol. Res.* 2011.

[5] Simoes B. M., Piva M., Iriondo O., et al. Effects of estrogen on the proportion of stem cells in the breast. *Breast Cancer Res. Treat.* 2011;129:23-35.

[6] Jordan V. C. The 38th David A. Karnofsky lecture: the paradoxical actions of estrogen in breast cancer--survival or death? *J. Clin. Oncol.* 2008;26:3073-82.

[7] Santen R. Estrogen hypersensitivity following estrogen deprivation. *Proc. Aromatase* 2000, Port Douglas 2000.

[8] Song R. X., Mor G., Naftolin F., et al. Effect of long-term estrogen deprivation on apoptotic responses of breast cancer cells to 17beta-estradiol. *J. Natl. Cancer Inst.* 2001;93:1714-23.

[9] Grady D., Rubin S. M., Petitti D. B., et al. Hormone therapy to prevent disease and prolong life in postmenopaUSl women [see comments]. *Ann. Intern. Med.* 1992;117:1016-37.

[10] Ragaz J., Coldman A. J. Age-matched all-cause mortality impact of hormone replacement therapy: applicability to breast cancer survivors. *Breast Ca Research and Treat.* 1999;57:30.

[11] Grodstein F., Stampfer M. J., Colditz G. A., et al. PostmenopaUSl hormone therapy and mortality. *N. Engl. J. Med.* 1997;336:1769-75.

[12] Rossouw J. E., Anderson G. L., Prentice R. L., et al. Risks and benefits of estrogen plus progestin in healthy postmenopaUSl women: principal results From the Women's Health Initiative randomized controlled trial. *Jama* 2002;288:321-33.

[13] Anderson G. L., Limacher M., Assaf A. R., et al. Effects of conjugated equine estrogen in postmenopaUSl women with hysterectomy: the Women's Health Initiative randomized controlled trial. *Jama* 2004;291:1701-12.

[14] Ravdin P. M., Cronin K. A., Howlader N., et al. The decrease in breast-cancer incidence in 2003 in the United States. *N. Engl. J. Med.* 2007;356:1670-4.

[15] Kuhl H. Effects of estrogen-only treatment in postmenopaUSl women.[comment]. *Jama* 2004;292:683; author reply 5-6.

[16] Rossouw J. E., Prentice R. L., Manson J. E., et al. PostmenopaUSl hormone therapy and risk of cardiovascular disease by age and years since menopause. *Jama* 2007;297:1465-77.

[17] Stefanick M. L., Anderson G. L., Margolis K. L., et al. Effects of conjugated equine estrogens on breast cancer and mammography screening in postmenopaUSl women with hysterectomy. *Jama* 2006;295:1647-57.

[18] Haddow A. David A. Karnofsky memorial lecture. Thoughts on chemical therapy. *Cancer* 1970;26:737-54.

[19] Boyer M. J., Tattersall M. H. Diethylstilbestrol revisited in advanced breast cancer management. *Med. Pediatr. Oncol.* 1990;18:317-20.

[20] Jordan V. C., Koerner S. Tamoxifen (ICI 46,474) and the human carcinoma 8S oestrogen receptor. *Eur. J. Cancer* 1975;11:205-6.

[21] Lippman M. E., Bolan G. Oestrogen-responsive human breast cancer in long term tissue culture. *Nature* 1975;256:592-3.

[22] Carter A. C., Sedransk N., Kelley R. M., et al. Diethylstilbestrol: recommended dosages for different categories of breast cancer patients. Report of the Cooperative Breast Cancer Group. *Jama* 1977;237:2079-8.

[23] Ellis M. J., Gao F., Dehdashti F., et al. Lower-dose vs high-dose oral estradiol therapy of hormone receptor-positive, aromatase inhibitor-resistant advanced breast cancer: a phase 2 randomized study. *Jama* 2009;302:774-80.

[24] Peethambaram P. P., Ingle J. N., Suman V. J., Hartmann L. C., Loprinzi C. L. Randomized trial of diethylstilbestrol vs. tamoxifen in postmenopaUSl women with metastatic breast cancer. An updated analysis. *Breast Cancer Res. Treat.* 1999;54:117-22.

[25] Ingle J. N., Ahmann D. L., Green S. J., et al. Randomized clinical trial of diethylstil-bestrol versus tamoxifen in postmenopaUSl women with advanced breast cancer. *N. Engl. J. Med.* 1981;304:16-21.

[26] Lewis-Wambi J. S., Jordan V. C. Estrogen regulation of apoptosis: how can one hormone stimulate and inhibit? *Breast Cancer Res.* 2009;11:206.

[27] Suba Z. Interplay Between Insulin Resistance and Estrogen Deficiency as co-Activators in Carcinogenesis. *Pathol. Oncol. Res.* 2012;18:123-33.

[28] Suba Z. Common soil of smoking-associated and hormone-related cancers: estrogen deficiency. *Oncology Reviews* 2010;4:73-87.

[29] Ragaz J., Le N., Budlovsky J., Spinelli J. Protective effect of estrogen (E2) and increased risk of E2 plus progestin (Prog) on breast cancer (BrCa). The 2009 review of the Women's Health Initiative (WHI) hormone replacement therapy (HRT) published trials. *Cancer Res.* 2009;69.

[30] Henderson I. C., Canellos G. P. Cancer of the breast: the past decade (first of two parts). *N. Engl. J. Med.* 1980;302:17-30.

[31] Henderson I. C., Canellos G. P. Cancer of the breast: the past decade (second of two parts). *N. Engl. J. Med.* 1980;302:78-90.

In: Estrogen Prevention for Breast Cancer
Editor: Zsuzsanna Suba

ISBN: 978-1-62417-378-3

Chapter VII

Failures and Controversies of the Antiestrogen Treatment of Breast Cancer

Zsuzsanna Suba

National Institute of Oncology, Department of Surgical and Molecular Pathology, Budapest, Hungary

Abstract

In postmenopausal women, estrogens have unquestionable preventive and curative effects against atherogenic cardiovascular lesions, osteoporosis and neurodegenerative diseases.

Moreover, recent studies on correlations between hormone replacement therapy and cancer risk could justify preventive, anticancer capacities of estrogen both on smoking associated and hormone related cancers.

Experimental developing of antiestrogen compounds aimed to inhibit the binding of presumably harmful, endogenous estrogen to its receptor system so as to achieve a regression of hormone-related cancers. However, antiestrogens proved to be ineffective in the majority of selected receptor positive breast cancer cases and produced severe side effects, such as vascular complications and cancer development at several sites. Failure of antiestrogen therapy was designated as "endocrine resistance" of tumors.

Therapeutic failures resulted in further search for effective drugs against hormone responsive tumors, designed as selective estrogen receptor modulators (SERMs). All these endocrine manipulations yielded fairly controversial results in breast cancer therapy, but the basic principle of estrogen carcinogenicity remained unquestionable. Moreover, a dangerous new trend is the recommendation of antiestrogens for cancer prevention at several sites.

Publications on the estrogen treatment of advanced breast cancer cases are regularly returning and the results are encouraging. Advantageous apoptotic effect of estrogen on advanced breast cancers was established as an adverse effect instead of proliferative activity.

Considering the newly introduced principle of the anticancer capacity of estrogen, the old-fashioned estrogen therapy in cancer treatment is to be applied and further developed.

Introduction

The idea of correlation between female sexual steroids and breast cancer risk had emerged more than 100 years ago based on empirical findings. Breast cancer was demonstrated to exhibit remission after ovariectomy in premenopausal women [1]. However, postmenopausal women occurred also frequently among breast cancer cases and this was strikingly explained by their abnormally elevated endogenous estrogen levels [2].

Hormone replacement therapy (HRT) against postmenopausal complaints of women became widespread in the past decades, especially in the economically developed countries [3]. Its use provided an excellent possibility to study the correlations between estrogen and breast cancer risk. Increasing prevalence of breast and endometrial cancers in Northern Europe and in the US seemed to be in close correlation with the popularity of HRT use. Results of subsequent studies in the past century suggested that breast, endometrial and ovarian cancers are hormonally induced tumors [4]. Both endogenous and exogenous elevated estrogen levels were presumed to play an important role in the development and progression of these cancers [5]. Carcinogenic capacity of estrogen has become a popular scientific field both for clinicians and researchers up to now. However, recent clinical studies revealed unexplained, beneficial anticancer effects of HRT use against oral, esophageal, gastric, colorectal, cervical, liver and lung cancer [6,7,8,9,10,11].

In the meantime, synthetic and natural estrogens were developed as therapeutic agents and their application has unique and indispensable possibilities in women, such as provocation of ovulation, and contraception in premenopausal cases. In postmenopausal women, estrogens have unquestionable preventive and curative effects against atherogenic cardiovascular lesions, osteoporosis and neurodegenerative diseases [12]. Moreover, recent studies on correlations between HRT and cancer risk could justify preventive, anticancer capacities of estrogen, even against the cancers of highly hormone responsive organs [13,14,15,16,17].

Protective effect of parity against breast cancer is well established [18]. In animal experiments pregnancy equivalent levels of estradiol were highly effective in the prevention of mammary, colorectal and kidney cancer induced by carcinogenic compounds [19,20,21].

Experimental development of antiestrogen compounds aimed to inhibit the binding of presumably harmful, endogenous estrogen to its receptor system so as to achieve a regression of hormone-related cancers. Tamoxifen was the first, clinically available antiestrogen proposed for cancer treatment [22]. However, antiestrogens proved to be ineffective in the majority of selected, estrogen receptor (ER) positive breast cancer cases and produced severe side effects, such as vascular complications and cancer development at several sites. Failure of antiestrogen therapy was designated as "endocrine resistance" of tumors [23].

Therapeutic failures resulted in further search for effective drugs against hormone responsive tumors, designed as selective estrogen receptor modulators (SERMs). These compounds were thought to be ideal to block the special signal transduction pathways of estrogen in cancer cells so as to achieve a tumor regression and to avoid side effects.

Aromatase inhibitors compose a further group of antiestrogen compounds, which blocks the enzyme converting androgens and other steroids to estrogen in ovaries and extraovarian tissues. Expectations to achieve a complete estrogen deprivation without harmful agonistic estrogen effects yielded further disappointment because of an unreliable inhibition of tumor growth and severe side effects [24].

All these endocrine manipulations yielded fairly controversial results in breast cancer therapy. Moreover, a dangerous new trend is the recommendation of antiestrogens for cancer prevention at several sites, in spite of their unreliable effect and severe, even life threatening side effects [12].

Estrogen treatment of tumors also emerged as breast cancer therapy in advanced cases. Publications on this therapeutic method applied in advanced breast cancer cases are regularly returning and they report on fairly encouraging results [25,26,27]. Many authors tried to explain the inverse, beneficial anticancer effect of the presumably carcinogenic estrogen. Advantageous apoptotic effects of high dose estrogen on advanced breast cancers were achieved in human therapy and it was evaluated as an adverse effect instead of proliferative activity [28,29].

This review will discuss the diverse molecular mechanisms of estrogen action and the controversial associations between estrogen effect and cancer initiation. Considering the newly introduced principle of the anticancer capacity of estrogen the therapeutic possibilities of antiestrogen and estrogen therapy in cancer treatment will also be analyzed.

Molecular Mechanisms of Estrogen Action

Role of estrogen and its receptors in gene regulation are thoroughly studied [30,31,32,33]. Review of literary data on the molecular mechanism of estrogen action suggests that estrogen orchestrates the gene regulation of cell proliferation with high safety [30,31,32]. Cross talk of estrogen receptors with other hormonal and growth factor signals, their agonistic and antagonistic interplay with other gene regulators suggest an indispensable role of estrogen in cell biology. However, estrogen deficiency may elicit a breakdown of the exquisite surveillance of gene regulation and results in disorders in cell proliferation beyond retrieval.

Gene regulation mechanisms affected by estrogen have a fairly wide range during pregnancy, embryonic growth, development and differentiation, and have a crucial role in the hormonal and metabolic processes both in males and females throughout the life. Estrogen, based on its pivotal role in gene regulation, has been accused of its carcinogenicity. However, as estrogen is a proven commander in chief in the regulation of endocrine functions, immune system, metabolism, and cell proliferation an extreme safeguarding is necessary to have domination over these highly responsible mechanisms.

Estrogen Receptors and Their Actions

In 1962 an estrogen binding receptor protein had been identified from rat uterus, which was supposed to mediate all actions of estrogen [34]. More than three decades later, in 1996 another isoform of estrogen receptor (ER) was discovered and named as ER-β [35], whereas the former ER was renamed as ER-α. These ER isoforms are the products of two distinct genes located on distinct chromosomes [36].

ERs belong to the steroid-thyroid hormone nuclear receptor superfamily [37]. The classic, genomic mechanism of ER action is that estrogen binding activates ERs in the nucleus and they act as transcriptional modulators by binding to specific sequences in the promoter region of target genes [32,38]. However, other signaling pathways that deviate from the classical model have been discovered, and recently it has been accepted that ERs regulate gene expression by a number of distinct mechanisms [32].

ERs can also regulate gene expression without direct binding to DNA, which occurs through interactions between receptor protein and other DNA-binding transcription factor proteins in the nucleus [32]. This interaction between ERs and transcription factors may result in either stimulation or inhibition in gene transcription processes [37]. Moreover, by means of some not clearly identified mechanisms, ERs may regulate the expression of genes that do not contain estrogen responsive elements (EREs).

Evidences are accumulating that estrogen action have also non-genomic, membrane associated signaling cascades [31]. Non-genomic actions may influence both the protein functions as a cytoplasmic network of coordination and the regulation of gene expression in the nucleus. Non-genomic actions are exerted by membrane associated ERs. Controversial concepts have been published concerning the nature of ERs located at the plasma membrane. Some authors have suggested that the non-genomic estrogen effects are mediated through a subpopulation of the classical two ER isoforms [39].

Finally, genomic and non-genomic pathways of estrogen receptor signaling converge on the target genes [32]. Several signal transduction pathways may connect the non-genomic estrogen actions to genomic responses. Many nuclear transcription factors are regulated through non-genomic protein kinase mediated phosphorylation, and these transcription factors may thus become targets for non-genomic estrogen actions. This complex signaling system provides an exquisitely safety control and plasticity of tissue responses to estrogen and also contributes to the divergence of tissue-specific actions [31].

ER-α is widely expressed throughout the female genital organs, such as in the uterus, vagina, ovaries and mammary glands, whereas it is also highly exhibited in the brain, bone, liver and cardiovascular system [40].

ER-β has been shown to be the dominant isoform in the prostate, testis, salivary glands, ovary, vascular endothelium, smooth muscle, certain neurons and in the cells of immune system [41]. Estrogen receptors in immune competent cells enable estrogen to regulate defense mechanisms against inflammatory processes, infections, shock and even malignant transformation.

Some tissues, such as mammary glands, uterus, brain, bone and cardiovascular system express both ER isoforms, with the predominance of one or the other [37,41]. All these sites are especially endangered in postmenopausal women with decreased ovarian hormone production. Incidence of ischemic attacks in the central nervous system, osteoporosis and dyslipidemic cardiovascular diseases is conspicuously increased in estrogen deficient female cases after menopause. In these diseases estrogen therapy has more or less beneficial effects, especially in the initial phases. Dangers of estrogen loss related to the breast and endometrium are newly recognized [13].

Presence of both alpha and beta ER isoforms was confirmed in adipocytes deriving from the subcutaneous and intra-abdominal location with evident predominance of ER-α [42]. Fatty tissue accumulation is fairly dependent on the equilibrium of sexual steroid levels. Estrogen tends to promote the gluteofemoral fat deposition [43], whereas estrogen loss and androgen excess is associated with abdominal obesity and strongly increases the risk of insulin resistance [44].

Postmenopausal aromatase activity and estrogen production in the adipose tissue have important role in many biological processes [45]. Recently, adipocytes have been regarded as endocrine cells. Fatty tissue is hormone dependent and in animal models hormones and cytokines produced by adipocytes have actions in remote organs, such as liver, muscle, bone, central nervous system and others [46]. Human adipose tissue and its secreted products have important role in the hormonal and metabolic processes. Hormonal regulation of human adipocytes may serve as a cross road among obesity, hypertension and insulin resistance [47].

ERs display similar DNA- and ligand binding properties in vitro, however, ER-β shows lower transcriptional activity than ER-α. Experimental results revealed that in the absence of estradiol both type of ERs interacted with estrogen responsive elements (EREs) in the nucleus similarly. However, estradiol application enhanced the ERE binding of ER-α but not that of ER-β. Thus, the interaction between ER-β and ERE seemed to be independent of estradiol and could be impaired by its amino terminus [48]. These findings provided additional explanation for differences between ER-α and ER-β actions. Moreover, these data also reveal that estrogen loss may yield thorough changes in gene expression mechanisms.

Summarizing the literary data, estradiol action depends on the ratio of receptor isoforms expressed in the given tissue. Moreover, in case of the coexpression of two receptors, interactions of their signaling pathways will variably modulate the transcription of target genes [33]. Great variations in tissular distribution and isoform predominance of ERs have been a source of intense debate among researchers. However, a widely accepted concept is that though ER-α and ER-β have distinct biological functions supposedly they act in a close interplay.

These overwhelming routes of estrogen effects and ER actions support that estrogen may use many different signaling pathways and will evoke distinct gene responses depending on the types of target cells and on the nature of temporary intra- and extracellular stimuli.

Interplay between Alpha and Beta Estrogen Receptor Isoforms in the Regulation of Cell Proliferation and of Apoptotic Cell Death

Mitogenic effect of estrogen is well known and thoroughly investigated, especially in context of cancer initiation and progression. Principle of the hormonal contribution of estrogen to carcinogenesis is based on its physiologic functions in gene regulation by means of its nuclear and plasma membrane receptors [49].

Estrogen receptor isoforms (ERα and ERβ) differently regulate epithelial cell proliferation and apoptotic cell death in normal tissues [50]. Different actions of ER-α and ER-β were observed on neuroblastoma cells transfected with either ER-α or ER-β. Activation of ER-α caused an increase in length and number of neurites, whereas ER-β activation resulted only in neurite elongation [51].

Discovery of selective agonists for ER-α and ER-β brought new possibilities to research the specificity of estrogen receptors. In an epithelial cell line obtained from pregnant mouse mammary glands both ER-α and ER-β was expressed. It was observed that selective agonists for ER-α provoke cell proliferation and agonists for ER-β inhibit cell growth on this in vitro model [50]. These findings suggest that a functional equilibrium of these two receptor isoforms may supply excellent surveillance for cell growth, differentiation and proliferation.

Development of the three knockout mouse lines: estrogen receptor-α and β knockout (ER-αKO, ER-βKO) [52] and aromatase enzyme knockout (ARKO) mice provided new opportunities for understanding the individual actions of the two estrogen receptors and of estrogen itself. In vivo studies on these knockout mice have demonstrated that ER-α and ER-β may have distinct, even opposite effects. Development of distinct autoimmune diseases in different knockout mice revealed that ER-α and ER-β have specific functions in the maintenance of normal immune system [33,53,54].

In addition to the specific function of each receptor, interplay between these two receptor isoforms has been reported when they are coexpressed. ER-β may oppose ER-α-mediated activity in many systems, moreover, ER-α and ER-β together may elicit completely opposite responses in the presence of estradiol [38,55]. In ER-βKO mice, ER-α-mediated gene expression was increased by 85% as compared with animals expressing both receptors. This observation suggested that ER-β in normal mice reduces ER-α-regulated gene transcription, supporting the idea of a “ying yang” relationship between the two receptors [56].

However, considering the magnitude, complexity and safety of estrogen receptor signals, actions of ER-α and ER-β can be hardly imagined as a mechanical equilibrium of a seesaw. Though there are multiple cross talks and interplays between the two ER isoforms, both of them may have their autoregulation with a simultaneous feedback control of the actions of other one. ER knockout mice are artificially disabled animals and similar disorders may occur extremely rarely as spontaneous mutations. Unexpected, increased gene expression elicited by the singly remaining ER-α may probably be attributed to an emergency substitution of the action of missing ER-β isoform.

Signal transduction and cross talk of these receptors provide a safety, momentary equilibrium of cell growth and mitotic activity defined by tissue type, functional activity and environmental influences. Both receptors bind 17β-estradiol (E2) with similar affinity; however, they can activate certain promoters differentially [57]. Moreover, on some promoter ERβ can behave as an inhibitor of ERα activity [58], and being aware of their mutual regulatory capacity ERα is also capable to block ERβ.

Physiological resistance to E2 induced cell proliferation was observed in mouse mammary cell line, HC11, which reflects the situation of late pregnant and lactating state of mammary glands [59]. Although these cells expressed both estrogen receptors they showed no proliferative activity.

These findings underline that expression of any receptor is not equal with its proliferative impact. A suggested mechanism responsible for resistance to E2-induced proliferation may be the reduction in coactivators and increase in corepressors [50]. Interplay between the activities of ER isoforms may explain that a concomitant activation of ERα and ERβ may equalize the opposing cellular responses regarding proliferation and apoptosis.

Both ERα and ERβ selective ligands were administered independently and effects exerted by one or the other receptor isoform were studied. PPT, an ERα-selective agonist provoked an increase in cell number nearly 50%, while DPN, an ERβ selective ligand caused a decrease of 30%. In neuroblastoma cells ERα agonist increased cell division and ERβ agonist provoked cell growth [50]. Both selective ligands had positive effects on cell metabolism as measured by dehydrogenase activity. Activation of each receptor alone increased cell metabolism independently as either mitotic activity or cell growth requires increase in cellular metabolism. However, the activation of both receptors simultaneously, either by E2 or by PPT-DPN combination produced equilibrium without increased metabolic activity.

The proliferative effects of E2 are mediated not only by transcriptional activation from ERE promoters but also by interactions of ERs with AP-1 binding proteins via protein-protein interactions [60]. Nevertheless, the ER signal transduction pathways affecting the cell proliferation are highly and diversely regulated and the mechanistic assumption regarding the exclusively opposing activities of ERα and ERβ are not completely justifiable. Results of experimental studies applying either alpha or beta ER agonists do not reflect physiological processes.

Cell proliferation is not an isolated process being quite independent of metabolic, hormonal and immunologic regulation. Protein, lipid and carbohydrate synthesis, mitochondrial activation, cell growth and their control by hormonal signals (e.g. growth hormone) are the predecessors of normal mitotic activity [61]. Estrogen and ER signals are essential players to harmonize the regulation of all these cellular functions. Separated activation or blocking of each ER isoforms may produce thorough alterations and disturbances in these processes. For example, ERα-knockout mice show severe insulin resistance [50]. This finding suggests that isolated block of ERα activity may have inhibitory effect on cell division but provokes metabolic disturbances, which will increase both cancer initiation and progression. Similarly, apoptotic effect of isolated ERβ activation is associated with insulin resistance and oxidative stress.

Presumably, there are two main estrogen-activated pathways, that is, proliferation by ERα and apoptotic cell death by ERβ [50]. Activation of both pathways by estrogen may be responsible for a dynamic equilibrium of cell number. In a non-malignant cell line the ratio of ERα to ERβ expression in cells may determine whether estradiol will induce proliferation or not [50]. However, forced separation of the activity of two ER isoforms will cause a breakdown of regulation even in healthy tissues and further disturbances in tumors without beneficial anticancer effects.

Embryonic development justifies the necessity of all ambiguous actions of estrogen. High estrogen levels in pregnant women ensure both explosion-like cell proliferation and the cessation of mitotic activity.

To date there is no consensus on the role of ERβ in breast cancer development [62]. In ER-positive breast cancers ERα mRNA was shown to be upregulated, whereas ERβ was downregulated. Other studies analyzed ERα and ERβ protein expression in normal breast tissue and histopathologically distinct breast lesions of different prognostic risk [63]. Important role of tissue concentration, relative expression and interaction of these two ER isoforms was established in modulating mammary tumor genesis.

ERβ expression was significantly decreased in breast cancer samples and metastatic lymph node tissues as compared with healthy mammary tissues [64]. Loss of ERβ expression could be one of the events involved in the development of colon cancer [65]. ERβ specific agonists might be candidates for treatment of some cancers [50,66]. Predominance of ERβ in highly differentiated tumors with preserved signal transduction pathways is a possibility for an induction of apoptotic cell death in estrogen-rich environment.

All these associations suggest that the overwhelming complexity of the transduction signal of estrogen receptors cannot be completely understood as our current knowledge probably covers only a small segment of their capacities. It is quite impossible to interfere with or even improve this highly controlled safeguard of estrogen on cellular mechanisms.

Considering the complex anticancer capacity of estrogen there is no sense to produce alternative compounds for the selective inhibition of its presumed "carcinogenic" activity with the preservation of beneficial estrogen effects.

Cross Talk between Receptor Signals of Estrogen and Growth Factors

Non-genomic actions of estrogen are too rapid to be attributed to RNA activation and protein synthesis. These actions are common properties of steroid hormones and are frequently associated with the activation of various protein-kinase cascades [67]. By these ways ERs have thorough surveillance on cell proliferation, which is their basic function during growth, differentiation and whole cell life.

Membrane associated ERs may activate membrane tyrosine kinase receptors in various cell types. ER-α activated by estradiol interacts directly with insulin-like growth factor-I (IGF-I) receptor, leading to its activation [68], and hence the activation of mitogen associated protein kinase (MAPK) signaling pathway [69]. These data demonstrate that estradiol activated ER-α is required for the rapid activation of IGF-I receptor signaling cascade.

Estradiol liganded ERs in the plasma membrane can rapidly stimulate signal transductions that are G-protein coupled. This was reported to occur through the transactivation of the epidermal growth factor receptor (EGFR) or insulin-like growth factor-I receptor (IGF-IR) [39]. Estrogen can overregulate the IGF-I gene transcription by involving an AP-I enhancer [68].

Estrogen signaling is coupled to growth factor signaling with a feedback mechanism directly impacting the function of growth factor receptors [30]. ER signaling pathways involving specific complexes of cytoplasmic proteins might either quench or augment the growth factor activities! On the other hand, the mitogen activated protein kinase system (MAPK) is capable of the phosphorylation of human estrogen receptor in vitro, and in cells treated with epidermal growth factor (EGF) and insulin like growth factor (IGF) in vivo. Thus the activity of the amino-terminal AF-l of ER may be modulated by the phosphorylation of Ser118 via the Ras-MAPK cascade of growth factor signaling pathways [70].

Estrogen dependent response in the uterus and mammary gland involves estradiol specific responses as well as responses resulting from a convergence of growth factor and ER-initiated activities [71,72].

Studies in rodents have shown that EGF is able to mimic the uterotropic effects of estrogen suggesting a physiological coupling of growth factor and steroid receptor signaling pathways. These results supplied a "cross-talk" model in which EGF receptor signaling resulted in activation of nuclear ERs [73]. However, in ER knockout mice epidermal growth factor could not elicit estrogen-like response, which revealed that intact ERs are necessary for the activation of ER target genes by growth factors [74].

In the absence of ER-ligand, the activators of protein kinase A or inhibitors of protein phosphatases are able to stimulate ER-dependent gene expression. Both EGF and IGF-I may stimulate the transcriptional activity of ERs in an estrogen independent manner. Cross talk between ERs and membrane receptors for growth factors may have physiological role in an estrogen deficient environment [75].

Estrogen has a crucial role in the regulation of growth hormone receptor (GHR) activities as well [61]. Estrogen attenuates growth hormone (GH) action by means of inhibition of its secretion and suppression of cellular GHR functions. Estrogen and GH concentrations are strongly correlated during puberty and later, in adult life GH levels are regularly higher in women than in men. In man the stimulatory effect of androgens on GH secretion depends on the ratio of their prior aromatisation to estrogens. All these observations suggest that estrogens play a major and positive role in the regulation of GH-IGF-I axis in both genders [61], which may be in close correlation with their antidiabetogenic and anticancer capacities.

Estrogen Receptors and Human Cancers

There are literary data on the supposed roles of estrogen and membrane-associated ER signaling pathways in human cancer induction [76,77], particularly in breast cancer cases [78,79,80].

Interactions of estrogen and growth factor receptors have been recently revealed in breast, lung and cholangial cancers [81,82]. In the majority of in vitro experiments on different tumor cell lines a close synergism of expressed estrogen and growth factor receptors was supposed in the modulation of cell growth and proliferation.

In human breast epithelial cells both growth inhibition and growth stimulation by estradiol were observed depending on the rate of ERs and GFRs. Moreover, the expression of epidermal growth factor receptor and estrogen receptor is often inversely correlated in human breast cancer cells [83].

Estrogen treatment could inhibit lung carcinogenesis by reducing levels of IGF-I [84], which is a potent mitogenic agent for several malignancies, including lung cancer. These results suggest rather an alternative role of estrogen and growth factor actions on tumor cell proliferation.

Role of estrogens in the development of lung cancer has been suggested as ERs were demonstrated in non-small cell lung cancers. In recent studies a favorable prognosis for patients with non-small cell lung cancer was established, when tumor cells exhibited increased expression of ERβ [85,86]. By contrast, the absence of Erβ nuclear staining correlated with poor survival in both men and women with lung cancer [87]. Associations of increased ERβ expression with a better prognosis of non-small cell lung cancer suggest an anticancer capacity of estrogen signal and raise the idea of beneficial effect of estrogen administration. This assumption seems to be justified by a recent study, which established a significant correlation between hormone replacement therapy and reduced lung cancer risk in postmenopausal women [11].

Highly expressed epidermal growth factor receptors were demonstrated in a variety of solid tumors, including oral cancer, and their activity enhanced the tumor growth and invasive capacity [88]. However, the role of estrogen effect in oral cancer development is not clearly understood. Estrogen receptor expression in oral cancers showed no correlation either with tumor progression or the mortality of patients [89]. Further studies indicated that cross talk between ERs and EGFRs means a common contribution to the development and progression of squamous cell cancer in head and neck region [90]. Nevertheless the presumed synergistic carcinogenic capacity of ERs and EGFRs would be a constant danger for cancer initiation without contraregulatory impact.

Aromatase inhibitors, which lower the estrogen ligand for ER and pure ER antagonists, which destroy the receptor, are used to cure breast cancer. Recently, recognition of a dynamic, inverse relationship between the expression of ERs and EGFRs has brought more excitement [83]. In apparently ER-negative breast cancer cells, a potential restoring of ER expression emerged by inhibition of growth factor signaling to overcome resistance to endocrine therapy [91]. Abandonment of estrogen deprivation and antiestrogen therapy in breast cancer cases should be more advantageous against growth factors instead of the idea of combined antiestrogen and anti-growth factor therapy.

Inhibition of vascular endothelial growth factor (VEGF) expression by ER-α exhibited in HEClA endometrial cancer cell line [92]. This finding suggests that the inhibition of capillary proliferation in tumors may be an important part of the anticancer capacity of ERs.

Estrogen receptor signal is thoroughly defended from the changes of serum estrogen levels by compensatory feedback mechanisms even in tumors. This suggests that elevated estrogen level may hardly produce gene alterations. Excessive estradiol treatment decreased the ER protein quantity in MCF-7 human breast cancer cell line within a few hours [93]. Similarly, estrogen administration evoked a decrease in ER-α protein and estrogen responsiveness in rat pituitaries [94]. On the other hand, in experimental animals the low serum estrogen levels increased the mRNA level of ERs [95]. This strict feedback regulation suggests that ER overexpression in highly estrogen responsive cells means an increased estrogen demand induced by estrogen deficiency rather than defense against excessive hormone supply.

Estrogen and growth factors are potent mitogenic stimuli that share important competitive capacities in the control of cell proliferation. Cross talk between ER and growth factor signals assures finical equilibrium and may result in either synergistic or antagonistic effects on gene regulation. Exquisitely organized genomic and non-genomic actions of ERs and their convergence on the target genes rather serve as a defense of gene regulation with a safety surveillance of multitude players in cell biology than as risk for malignancy.

In the absence of estrogens, the biological equilibrium of gene regulation is endangered. There is no estrogen to exert its indispensable cellular actions and to oppose overwhelming growth factor activities. Accumulation of non-liganded ERs in estrogen deficient milieu may also result in emergency coupling of GF and ER signals resulting in a compensatory activation of nuclear ERs. Moreover, excessive IGF-I and EGF signals might modulate the functions of exposed, non-liganded ERs through their phosphorylation on certain residues [30]. These might be dangerous processes as unopposed growth factor activities and the altered phosphorylation of non liganded ERs may provoke a blunder in the gene regulation of cell proliferation. Breakdown in the main regulatory signals may result in cancer initiation [96].

Estrogen Synthesis in Tumors

Recently, postmenopausal estrogen production has been justified in the cells of different organs with high estrogen demand [33]. Aromatase activity and estrogen synthesis in the endothelium, glia, bone, breast and endometrium evoked many controversies and debates. Some authors regarded estrogen accumulation in the breast tissue of postmenopausal women as a justification of hormone induced carcinogenesis in spite of a decreased circulatory estrogen level [97]. However, this extraovarian estrogen synthesis may be a defensive mechanism for organs, which exhibit enhanced vulnerability in estrogen deficient environment rather than a possibility to access chronic diseases, even cancers in postmenopausal cases.

In situ synthesis of estrogens by breast cancer tissue provided potential explanation for high estradiol concentrations in the mammary neoplasms of postmenopausal women [98]. Moreover, in breast cancer cases a local estrogen production of carcinoma cells, stromal cells and adipocytes adjacent to the tumor was justified by abundantly expressed aromatase enzyme activity [99]. Intratumoral aromatase activity and increased in situ estrogen concentration were particularly demonstrated at the invasive front of cancers where the tumor-stromal interactions may define the spread of cancer cells [100].

Considering the concept of the anticancer capacity of estrogen, this hormone synthetizing interaction between cancer and stromal cells may be evaluated rather as a defense mechanism against tumor invasion at the hot zone. Estrogen synthesis by stromal cells and adipocytes adjacent to the invasive front of cancer may be regarded as a defensive host reaction against tumor spread.

On the contrary, the estrogen-producing capacity of highly differentiated breast cancer cells seems to be a kamikaze action. Taken into account the consequent ER positivism of highly differentiated, slowly growing breast tumors, they may preserve the aromatase activity and thus the estrogen synthetizing capacity of their mother tissue. Estrogen production of highly differentiated, ER-positive breast cancer cells may explain their slow tumor spread and the long lasting survival of patients with such tumors.

Antiestrogen and Estrogen in Cancer Therapy

Tamoxifen was originally designated as an antiestrogen compound, which selectively binds to estrogen receptors inhibiting their signal pathways. It is widely used as an adjuvant therapy for early stage ER positive breast cancers. However, the benefits of this antiestrogen compound are not equivocal in cancer therapy [24].

Even among women with ER positive breast cancers only 40-50% of patients exhibit primarily successful tumor regression [101]. These results suggest that more than half of ER positive breast cancers are de novo resistant to this endocrine therapy (102). A large proportion of earlier responsive breast cancers may acquire secondary resistance during tamoxifen therapy resulting in tumor progression and death [103]. Moreover, tamoxifen may elicit common side effects, which maybe occasionally life threatening [103,104,105,106]. Increased prevalence of stroke, pulmonary emboli and malignancies at several sites associated with tamoxifen administration has been surprisingly attributed to its preserved estrogenic activity [23].

Explanation for this high rate of therapeutic failures designated as "resistance" may be that tamoxifen is regarded rather a selective estrogen receptor modulator (SERM) with variable agonistic and antagonistic activities. Its effects fairly depend on the distribution and ratio of ER-alpha and ER-beta expression in the tumors and on further factors influencing receptor binding [107]. In therapy resistant ER positive breast cancers tamoxifen is thought to behave like an estrogen similarly as it is presumed in bone, liver and coronary arteries, rather than an antiestrogen [108,109]. Taking tamoxifen for either SERM or antiestrogen, unsuccessful treatment on more than the half of selected patients with receptor positive breast cancer exactly defines its therapeutic failure.

Though there are overwhelming advances in understanding the signal pathways of ERs [132] their cross talks and interplays with epidermal growth factor receptors (EGFRs) and insulin-like growth factor receptors (IGFRs) hide many obscure details [110]. These correlations have undoubtedly essential role in the stimulation and inhibition of tumor growth. Being aware of the highly regulated ER signals even in differentiated tumors and supposing a mixture of agonistic and antagonistic impacts of SERMs it is impossible to prophecy, which signal pathways will be stimulated or inhibited.

Further group of antiestrogens is known as aromatase inhibitors, which prevent the activity of P450 aromatase [24]. This enzyme converts steroid precursors and androgens to estradiol both in healthy tissues and tumors and its inhibition means estrogen deprivation. Clinical investigations have demonstrated that aromatase inhibitors are at least as effective, or even better than tamoxifen. However, they have severe side effects related to estrogen depletion, such as osteoporosis and spontaneous bone fractures. By the introduction of aromatase inhibitors as therapeutic agents the supposed estrogen agonist activities of SERMs are successfully avoided but their anticancer effects are insufficient.

Being aware of the anticancer capacity of ER signal, estrogen deprivation caused by aromatase inhibitors seems to be less harmful as compared with tamoxifen, which destroys ERs.

Accidental tumor inhibitory effect of antiestrogens can be explained by several ways. In case of availability of intact ERs there are possibilities for getting estrogen signal over estrogen deprivation. Lower estrogen concentration may elicit a higher ER expression level by means of feedback mechanism, which may be a refugee for the endangered estrogen action [95]. Moreover, EGFR signal may also activate intact ERs by an accidental coupling of their signaling pathways so as to evoke an estrogen-like impact in emergency situation caused by estrogen deprivation [74]. By means of such complicated mechanisms estrogen signal makes its escape and may inhibit the tumor progression in spite of antiestrogen administration. Tamoxifen is a powerful inhibitor of mitochondrial electron transport chain and increase superoxide radical generation by its ER blocking activity [111], which are cytotoxic effects with possible anticancer capacity.

Results of widespread antiestrogen tumor treatment by SERMs seem to be ambiguous. These controversial data can be equally explained based on the principle of either the carcinogenic or anticancer capacity of estrogen. Considering the supposed carcinogenic capacity of estrogen, like Dr. Jekyll, tamoxifen may contribute to the tumor regression as a receptor antagonist. However, like Mr. Hyde, cloaked in the disguise of an agonist it is supposed to cause harmful tumor progression as well [101]. Recognition of the anticancer capacity of estrogen helps to evaluate tamoxifen in breast cancer therapy quite inversely. ER agonistic impact associated with tamoxifen use may be regarded as getting estrogen signal through its inhibition, which results in beneficial tumor regression. However, if estrogen signal is defeated by the ER antagonistic actions of tamoxifen it might provoke local and metastatic spread of breast cancers.

Cancer provoking impacts of antiestrogens are equivocally justified by the exhibition of malignancies as their side effects, such as endometrial and gastrointestinal cancers [23]. Nevertheless, one can hardly imagine that the same compound has exclusive therapeutic action on breast cancer and in the meantime induces further malignancies at several sites by means of binding to the same receptor system. As a matter of fact, antiestrogen is not an adequate choice for breast cancer therapy either in theory or in practice.

Alternatively, estrogen therapy was also introduced as a possibility in breast cancer treatment with promising results. High dose estrogen was successfully administered as endocrine therapy for postmenopaUSl women with advanced breast cancer before the introduction of tamoxifen [25,27]. Subsequently, the use of estrogen as anticancer therapy was near completely abandoned. Recently, the "old-fashioned" high-dose estrogen treatment in patients with advanced breast cancer and previous estrogen deprivation was demonstrated to be effective in prospective clinical trials [27]. Moreover, women with advanced breast cancer and acquired resistance to aromatase inhibitor therapy were successfully treated even by lower doses of oral estradiol as well [112]. Low dose estrogen therapy resulted in a markedly lower incidence of serious adverse effects and at the same time good tumor regression.

Anti-tumor mechanism of estrogen therapy remained unknown. Nevertheless, estrogen may become an apoptotic trigger rather than a survival signal after many years of estrogen deprivation [29,112]. One can hypothesize that long-term aromatase inhibitor treatment may sensitize the hormone receptor positive breast cancer cells even to a low dose estrogen therapy.

Conclusion

Successful treatment of patients with advanced breast tumors by estrogen administration seems to justify the anticancer capacity of estrogen. Nevertheless, the ambiguous, unreliable therapeutic effects and high toxicity of antiestrogens suggests the necessity of finding new strategies in cancer treatment instead of fighting against a presumed endocrine "resistance".

References

[1] Beatson T. G.: On the treatment of inoperable cases of carcinoma of the mamma. Suggestions for a new treatment with illustrative cases. *Lancet* 2:104-107, 1896.

[2] Berrino F., Muti P., Micheli A., Bolelli G., Krogh V., Sciajno R. et al: Serum sex hormone levels after menopause and subsequent breast cancer. *J. Natl. Cancer Inst.* 88:291-296, 1996.

[3] Grady D.: Postmenopausal hormones-therapy for symptoms only. *New Engl. J. Med.* 348:1-3, 2003.
[4] International Agency for Research on Cancer: Monographs on the evaluation of carcinogenic risks to humans: hormonal contraception and postmenopausal hormone therapy. Vol. 72. I. A. R. C., Lyon, 1999.
[5] Russo J., Ao X., Grill C., Russo I. H.: Pattern of distribution of cells positive for estrogen receptor-α and progesterone receptor in relation to proliferating cells in the mammary gland. *Breast Cancer Res. Treat* 53:217-227, 1999.
[6] La Vecchia C., Brinton L. A., McTiernan A.: Menopause, hormone replacement therapy and cancer. *Maturitas* 39:97-115, 2001.
[7] Fernandez E., Gallus S., Bosetti C., Franceschi S., Negri E., La Vecchia C.: Hormone replacement therapy and cancer risk: a systematic analysis from a network of case-control studies. *Int. J. Cancer* 105:408-412, 2003.
[8] Gallus S., Bosetti C., Franceschi S., Levi F., Simonato L., Negri E., La Vecchia C.: Oesophageal cancer in women: tobacco, alcohol, nutritional and hormonal factors. *Br. J. Cancer* 85:341-345, 2001.
[9] Olsson H., Bladström A. M., Ingvar C.: Are smoking-associated cancers prevented or postponed in women using hormone replacement therapy? *Obstet. Gynecol.* 102:565–570, 2003.
[10] Parazzini F., La Vecchia C., Negri E., Franceschi S., Bolis G.: Case-control study of estrogen replacement therapy and risk of cervical cancer. *Br. Med. J.* 315:85-88, 1997.
[11] Rodriguez C., Feigelson H. S., Deka A., Patel A. V., Jacobs E. J., Thun M. J., Calle E. E.: Postmenopausal hormone therapy and lung cancer risk in the Cancer Prevention Study II Nutrition Cohort. *Cancer Epidemiol. Biomarkers Prev.* 17:655-660, 2008.
[12] Ascenzi P., Bocedi A., Marino M.: Structure-function relationship of estrogen receptor alpha and beta: impact on human health. *Mol. Aspects Med.* 27:299-402, 2006.
[13] Suba Zs: Common soil of smoking-associated and hormone-related cancers: estrogen deficiency. *Oncol. Rev.* 4:73-87, 2010.
[14] Suba Zs: Re-evaluation of the epidemiological associations of female sexual steroids and cancer risk, Chapter 6. pp. 108-125 In: Estrogen versus Cancer, Nova Science Publishers Inc, New York, 2009.
[15] Anderson G. L., Limacher M., Assaf A. R., Bassford T., Beresford S. A., Black H., Bonds D., Brunner R., Brzyski R., Caan B., Chlebowski R., Curb D., Gass M., Hays J., Heiss G., Hendrix S., Howard B. V., Hsia J., Hubbell A., Jackson R., Johnson K. C., Judd H., Kotchen J. M., Kuller L., LaCroix A. Z., Lane D., Langer R. D., Lasser N., Lewis C. E., Manson J., Margolis K., Ockene J., O'Sullian M. J., Phillips L., Prentice R. L., Ritenbaugh C., Robbins J., Rossouw J. E., Sarto G., Stefanick M. L., Van Horn L., Wactawski-Wende J., Wallace R., Wassertheil-Smoller S., Women's Health Initiative Steering Committee: Effects of conjugated equine estrogen in postmenopaUSl women with hysterectomy: the Women's Health Initiative randomized controlled trial. *J. A. M. A.* 291:1701–1712, 2004.
[16] Anderson G. L., Judd H. L., Kaunitz A. M. Women's Health Initiative Investigators: Effects of estrogen plus progestin on gynecologic cancers and associated diagnostic procedures: The Women's Health Initiative randomized trial. *J. A. M. A.* 290:1739-1748, 2003.

[17] Shapiro S.: False alarm: postmenopaUSl hormone therapy and ovarian cancer. *Climacteric* 10:466-470, 2007.

[18] Britt K., Ashworth A., Smalley M.: Pregnancy and the risk of breast cancer.*Endocrine-Related Cancer* 14:907-933, 2007.

[19] Rajkumar L., Guzman R. C., Yang J., Thordarson G., Talamantes F., Nandi S.: Prevention of mammary carcinogenesis by short-term estrogen and progestin treatments. *Breast Cancer Res.* 6:31-37, 2004.

[20] Smirnoff P., Liel Y., Gnainsky J., Shany S., Schwartz B.: The protective effect of estrogen against chemically induced murine colon carcinogenesis is associated with decreased CpG island methylation and increased mRNA and protein expression of the colonic vitamin D receptor. *Oncol. Res.* 11:255-264, 1999.

[21] Deguchi J., Miyamoto M., Okada S.: Sex hormone-dependent renal cell carcinogenesis induced by ferric nitrilotriacetate in Wistar rats. *Jpn. J. Cancer Res.* 86:1068-1071, 1995.

[22] Lerner L. J., Jordan V. C.: Development of antiestrogens and their use in breast cancer: eighth Cain memorial award lecture. *Cancer Res.* 50:4177-4189, 1990.

[23] Braithwaite R. S., Chlebowski R. T., Lau J., George S., Hess R., Col F. N.: Meta-analysis of vascular and neoplastic events associated with tamoxifen. *J. General Int. Med.* 18:937-947, 2003.

[24] Lin N. U., Winer E. P.: Advances in adjuvant endocrine therapy for postmenopausal women. *J. Clin. Oncol.* 26:798-805, 2008.

[25] Ingle J. N.: Estrogen as therapy for breast cancer. *Breast Cancer Res.* 4:133-136, 2002.

[26] Lønning P. E., Taylor P. D., Anker G., Iddon J., Wie L., Jørgensen L. M., Mella O., Howell A.: High-dose estrogen treatment in postmenopausal breast cancer patients heavily exposed to endocrine therapy. *Breast Cancer Res. Treat.* 67:111-116, 2001.

[27] Lønning P. E.: Additive endocrine therapy for advanced breast cancer; back to the future. *Acta Oncol.* 48:1092-1101, 2009.

[28] Jordan V. C., Lewis-Wambi J. S., Patel R. R., Kim H., Ariazi E. A.: New hypotheses and opportunities in endocrine therapy: amplification of estrogen-induced apoptosis. *Breast* 18:S10-S17, 2009.

[29] Maximov P. Y., Lewis-Wambi J. S., Jordan V. C., Knudson A. G.: The paradox of oestradiol-induced breast cancer cell growth and apoptosis. *Current Signal Transduct. Ther.* 4:88-102, 2009.

[30] Driggers P. H., Segars J. H.: Estrogen action and cytoplasmic signaling pathways. Part II: The role of growth factors and phosphorylation in estrogen signaling. *Trends Endocrin. Metab.* 13:422-427, 2002.

[31] Segars J., Driggers P.: Estrogen action and cytoplasmic signaling cascades. Part I: Membrane-associated signaling complexes. *Trends Endocrin. Metab.* 13:349-354, 2002.

[32] Björnström L., Sjöberg M.: Mechanisms of estrogen receptor signaling: Convergence of genomic and nongenomic actions on target genes. *Mol. Endocrinol.* 19:833-842, 2005.

[33] Barros R. P. A., Machado U. F., Gustafsson J. A.: Estrogen receptors: new players in diabetes mellitus. *Trends Molecular Med.* 9:425-431, 2006.

[34] Jensen E. V., Jacobson H. I.: Basic guides to the mechanism of estrogen action. *Recent Prog. Horm. Res.* 18:387-414, 1962.

[35] Kuiper G. G., Enmark E., Pelto-Huikko M., Nilsson S., Gustafsson J. A.: Cloning of a novel receptor expressed in rat prostate and ovary. *Proc. Natl. Acad. Sci. US* 93:5925-5930, 1996.

[36] Enmark E., Pelto-Huikko M., Grandien K., Lagercrantz S., Lagercrantz J., Fried G., Nordenskjold M., Gustafsson J. A.: Human estrogen receptor beta-gene structure, chromosomal localization and expression pattern. *J. Clin. Endocrinol. Metab.* 82:4258-4265, 1997.

[37] Nilsson S., Makela S., Treuter E., Tujague J., Thomsen J., Andersson G., Enmark E., Pettersson K., Warner M., Gustafsson J. A.: Mechanisms of estrogen action. *Physiol. Rev.* 81:1535-1565, 2001.

[38] Hall J. M., McDonnell D. P.: The estrogen receptor β-isoform (ERβ) of the human estrogen receptor modulates ERα transcriptional activity and is a key regulator of the cellular response to estrogens and antiestrogens. *Endocrinol.* 140:5566-5578, 1999.

[39] Razandi M., Pedram A., Greene G. L., Levin E. R.: Cell membrane and nuclear estrogen receptors (ERs) originate from a single transcript: studies of ERα and ERβ expressed in Chinese hamster ovary cells. *Mol. Endocrinol.* 13:307-319, 1999.

[40] Katzenellenbogen B. S.: Estrogen receptors: bioactivities and interactions with cell signaling pathways. *Biol. Reprod.* 54:287-293, 1996.

[41] Koehler K. F., Helguero L. A., Haldosen L. A., Warner M., Gustafsson J. A.: Reflections on the discovery and significance of estrogen receptor β. *Endocr. Rev.* 26:465-478, 2005.

[42] Dieudonne M. N., Leneveu M. C., Giudicelli Y., Pecquery R.: Evidence for functional estrogen receptors α and β in human adipose cells: regional specificies and regulation by estrogens. *Am. J. Physiol. Cell Physiol.* 286:C655-C661, 2004.

[43] Krotkiewski M., Björntorp P., Sjostrom L., Smith U.: Impact of obesity on metabolism in men and women, importance of regional adipose tissue distribution. *J. Clin. Invest.* 72: 1150-1162, 1983.

[44] Poehlman E. T., Toth M. J., Gardner A. W.: Changes in energy balance and body composition at menopause: a controlled longitudinal study. *Ann. Intern. Med.* 123:673-675, 1995.

[45] Judd H. I., Shamonki I. M., Frumar A. M., Lagasse L. D.: Origin of serum estradiol in postmenopausal women. *Obstet. Gynecol.* 59:680-686, 1982.

[46] Mattison R., Jensen M.: The adipocyte as an endocrine cell. *Curr. Opin. Endocrinol. Diab.* 10:317-321, 2003.

[47] Tikhonoff V., Staessen J. A.: Hormonal regulation of human adipocytes at the cross roads between obesity and hypertension. *J. Hypertens.* 20:839-841, 2002.

[48] Huang J., Li X., Maguire C. A., Hilf R., Bambara R. A., Muyan M.: Binding of estrogen receptor beta to estrogen response element in situ is independent of estradiol and impaired by its amino terminus. *Mol. Endocrinol.* 19:2696-2712, 2005.

[49] Dickson R. B., Gelmann E. P., Knabbe C., Jasid K., Bates S., Swain S.: Mechanisms of estrogenic and antiestrogenic regulation of growth of human breast carcinoma. In: Klijn J. G. M. (ed) *Hormonal manipulation of cancer: peptides, growth factors, and new (anti) steroidal agents.* Raven Press, New York, pp. 381-403, 1987.

[50] Helguero L. A., Faulds M. H., Gustafsson J. A., Haldosen L. A.: Estrogen receptors α (ERα) and β (ERβ) differentially regulate proliferation and apoptosis of the normal murine mammary epithelial cell line HC11. *Oncogene* 24:6605-6616, 2005.

[51] Patrone C., Pollio G., Vegeto E., Enmark E., de Curtis I., Gustafsson J. A., Maggi A.: Estradiol induces differential neuronal phenotypes by activating estrogen receptor α or β. *Endocrinol.* 141:1839-1845, 2000.

[52] Krege J. K., Hodgin J. B., Couse J. F., Enmark E., Warner M., Mahler J. F., Sar M., Korach K. S., Gustafsson J. A., Smithies O.: Generation and reproductive phenotypes of mice lacking estrogen receptor β. *Proc. Natl. Acad. Sci. US* 95:15677-15682, 1998.

[53] Shim G. J., Kis L. L., Warner M., Gustafsson J. A.: Autoimmune glomerulonephritis with spontaneous formation of splenic germinal centers in mice lacking the estrogen receptor α gene. *Proc. Natl. Acad. Sci. US* 101:1720-1724, 2004.

[54] Shim G. J., Warner M., Kim H. J., Andersson S., Liu L., Ekman J., Imamov O., Jones M. E., Simpson E. R., Gustafsson J. A.: Aromatase-deficient mice spontaneously develop a lymphoproliferative autoimmune disease resembling Sjögren's syndrome. *Proc. Natl. Acad. Sci. US* 101:12628-12633, 2004.

[55] Maruyama S., Fujimoto N., Asano K., Ito A.: Suppression by estrogen receptor β of AP-1 mediated transactivation through estrogen receptor α. *J. Steroid Biochem. Mol. Biol.* 78:177-184, 2001.

[56] Lindberg M. K., Moverare S., Skrtic S., Gao H., Dahlman-Wright K., Gustafsson J. A., Ohlsson C.: Estrogen receptor (ER)-β reduces ERα-regulated gene transcription, supporting a 'ying yang' relationship between ERα and ERβ in mice. *Mol. Endocrinol.* 17:203-208, 2003.

[57] Saville B., Wormke M., Wang F., Nguyen T., Enmark E., Kuiper G., Gustafsson J. A., Safe S.: Ligand-, cell-, and estrogen receptor subtype (alpha/beta)-dependent activation at GC-rich (Sp1) promoter elements. *J. Biol. Chem.* 275:5379-5387, 2000.

[58] Weihua Z., Andersson S., Cheng G., Simpson E. R., Warner M., Gustafsson J. A.: Update on estrogen signaling. *F. E. B. S. Letters* 546:17-24, 2003.

[59] Shyamala G., Ferenczy A.: The nonresponsiveness of lactating mammary gland to estradiol. *Endocrinol.* 110:1249-1256, 1982.

[60] Kushner P. J., Agard D. A., Greene G. L., Scanlan T. S., Shiau A. K., Uht R. M., Webb P.: Estrogen receptor pathways to AP-1. *J. Steroid Biochem. and Mol. Biol.* 74:311-317, 2000.

[61] Leung K. C., Johannson G., Leong G. M., Ho K. K. Y.: Estrogen regulation of growth hormone action. *Endocrine Rev.* 25:693-721, 2004.

[62] Fuqua S. A., Schiff R., Parra I., Moore J. T., Mohsin S. K., Osborne C. K., Clark G. M., Allred D. C.: Estrogen receptor beta protein in human breast cancer: correlation with clinical tumor parameters. *Cancer Res.* 63:2434-2439, 2003.

[63] Shaaban A. M., O'Neill P. A., Davies M. P., Sibson R., West C. R., Smith P. H., Foster C. S.: Declining estrogen receptor-beta expression defines malignant progression of human breast neoplasia. *Am. J. Surg. Pathol.* 27:1502-1512, 2003.

[64] Park B. W., Kim K. S., Heo M. K., Ko S. S., Hong S. W., Yang W. I., Kim J. H., Kim G. E., Lee K. S.: Expression of estrogen receptor-beta in normal mammary and tumor tissues: is it protective in breast carcinogenesis. *Breast Cancer Res. Treat.* 80:79-85, 2003.

[65] Martineti V., Picariello L., Tognarini I., Carbonell Sala S., Gozzini A., Azzari C., Mavilia C., Tanini A., Falchetti A., Fiorelli G., Tonelli F., Brandi M. L.: ER-beta is a potent inhibitor of cell proliferation in the HCT8 human colon cancer cell line through regulation of cell cycle components. *Endocrine-Related Cancer* 12:455-469, 2005.

[66] Pravettoni A., Mornati O., Martini P. G., Marino M., Colciago A., Celotti F., Motta M., Negri-Cesi P.: Estrogen receptor beta (ER-beta) and inhibition of prostate cancer cell proliferation: studies on the possible mechanism of action in DU145 cells. *Mol. Cell Endocrinol.* 263:46-54, 2007.

[67] Losel R., Wehling M.: Nongenomic actions of steroid hormones. *Nat. Rev. Mol. Cell Biol.* 4:46-56, 2003.

[68] Umayahara Y., Kawamori R., Watada H., Imano E., Iwama N., Morishima T., Yamasaki Y., Kajimoto Y., Kamada T.: Estrogen regulation of the insulin-like growth factor I gene transcription involves an AP-l enhancer. *J. Biol. Chem.* 269:16433-16442, 1994.

[69] Kahlert S., Neudling S., van Eickels M., Vetter H., Meyer R., Groche C.: Estrogen receptor α rapidly activates the IGF-1 receptor pathway. *J. Biol. Chem.* 275:18447-18453, 2000.

[70] Kato S., Endoh H., Masuhiro Y., Kitamoto T., Uchiyama S., Sasaki H., Masushige S., Gotoh Y., Nishida E., Kawashima H., Metzger D., Chambon P.: Activation of the estrogen receptor though phosphorylation by mitogen-activated protein kinase. *Science* 270: 1491-1494, 1995.

[71] Hewitt S. C., Collins J., Grissom S., Deroo B., Korach K. S.: Global uterine genomics in vivo: microarray evaluation of the estrogen receptor alpha-growth factor cross-talk mechanism. *Mol. Endocrinol.* 19:657-668, 2005.

[72] Ankrapp D. P., Bennett J. M., Haslam S. Z.: Role of epidermal growth factor in the acquisition of ovarian steroid hormone responsiveness in the normal mouse mammary gland. *J. Cell Physiol.* 174:251-260, 1998.

[73] Nelson K. G., Takahashi T., Bossert N. L., Walmer D. K., McLachlan J. A.: Epidermal growth factor replaces estrogen in the stimulation of female genital-tract growth and differentiation. *Proceed. Natl. Acad. Sci. US* 88:21-25, 1991.

[74] Curtis S. W., Washburn T., Sewall C., DiAugustine R., Lindzey J., Couse J. F., Korach K. S.: Physiological coupling of growth factor and steroid receptor signaling pathway: estrogen receptor knockout mice lack estrogen-like response to epidermal growth factor. P*roceed. Natl. Acad. Sci. US* 93: 12626-12630, 1996.

[75] Smith C. L.: Cross-talk between peptide growth factor and estrogen receptor signaling pathways. *Biol. Reprod.* 58:627-632, 1998.

[76] Henderson B. E., Ross R., Bernstein L.: Estrogens as a cause of human cancer. *Cancer Res.* 48:246-253, 1988.

[77] Pietras R. J., Marquez-Garban D. C.: Membrane-associated estrogen receptor signaling pathways in human cancers. *Clin. Cancer Res.* 13:4672-4676, 2007.

[78] Key T. J., Applyby P. N., Reeves G. K., Roddam A., Dorgan J. F., Longcope C., Stanczyk F. Z., Stephenson H. E. Jr, Falk R. T., Miller R., Schatzkin A., Allen D. S., Fentiman I. S., Key T. J.,Wang D. Y., Dowsett M., Thomas H. V., Hankinson S. E., Toniolo P., Akhmedkhanov A., Koenig K., Shore R. E., Zeleniuch-Jacquotte A., Berrino F., Muti P., Micheli A., Krogh V., Sieri S., Pala V., Venturelli E., Secreto G., Barrett-Connor E., Laughlin G. A., Kabuto M., Akiba S., Stevens R. G., Neriishi K.,

Land C. E., Cauley J. A., Kuller L. H., Cummings S. R., Helzlsouer K. J., Alberg A. J., Bush T. L., Comstock G. W., Gordon G. B., Miller S. R., Longcope C., Endogenous Hormones Breast Cancer Collaborative Group: Body mass index, serum sex hormones and breast cancer risk in postmenopausal women. *J. Natl. Cancer Inst.* 95: 1218-1226, 2003.

[79] Marquez D. C., Pietras R. J.: Membrane-associated binding sites for estrogen contribute to growth regulation in human breast cancer cells. *Oncogene* 20:5420-5430, 2001.

[80] Pietras R. J., Arboleda J., Wongvipat N., Ramos L., Parker M. G., Sliwkowski M. X., Slamon D. J.: HER-2 tyrosine kinase pathway targets estrogen receptor and promotes hormone independent growths in human breast cancer cells. *Oncogene* 10:2435-2446, 1995.

[81] Alvaro D., Barbaro B., Franchitto A., Onori P., Glaser S. S., Alpini G., Francis H., Marucci L., Sterpetti P., Ginanni-Corradini S., Onetti M. A., Dostal D. E., De Santis A., Attili A. F., Benedetti A., Gaudio E.: Estrogens and insulin-like growth factor I modulate neoplastic cell growth in human cholangiocarcinoma. *Am. J. Path.* 169:877-888, 2006.

[82] Pietras R. J., Marquez D., Chen H. W., Tsai E., Weinberg O., Fishbein M.: Estrogen and growth factor receptor interactions in human breast and non-small cell lung cancer cells. *Steroids* 70:372-381, 2005.

[83] Lundholt B. K., Briand P., Lykkesfeldt A. E.: Growth inhibition and growth stimulation by estradiol of estrogen receptor transfected human breast epithelial cell lines involve different pathways. *Breast Cancer Res. Treat.* 67:199-214, 2001.

[84] Marquez-Garban D. C., Chen H. W., Fishbein M. C., Goodglick L., Pietras R. J.: Estrogen receptor signaling pathways in human non-small cell lung cancer. *Steroids* 72:135-143, 2007.

[85] Skov B. G., Fischer B. M., Pappot H.: Oestrogen receptor beta over expression in males with non-small cell lung cancer is associated with better survival. *Lung Cancer* 59:88-94, 2008.

[86] Wu C. T., Chang Y. L., Shih J. Y., Lee Y. C.: The significance of estrogen receptor beta in 301 surgically treated non-small cell lung cancers. *J. Thorac Cardiovasc. Surg.* 130:979-986, 2005.

[87] Kaway H., Ishii A., Washiya K., Konno T., Kon H., Yamaya C., Ono I., Minamiya Y., Ogawa J.: Estrogen receptor alpha and beta are prognostic factors in non-small cell lung cancer. *Clin. Cancer Res.* 11:5084-5089, 2005.

[88] Hirashi Y., Wada T., Nakatani K., Negoro K., Fujita Sh: Immunohistochemical expression of EGFR and p-EGFR in oral squamous cell carcinomas. *Pathol. Oncol. Res. 12*:87-91, 2006.

[89] Lukits J., Remenar E., Raso E., Ladányi A., Kasler M., Timar J.: Molecular identification, expression and prognostic role of estrogen- and progesterone receptors in head and neck cancer. *Int. J. Oncol.* 30:155-160, 2007.

[90] Egloff A. M., Rothstein M. E., Seethala R., Siegfriend J. M., Grandis J. R., Stabile L. P.: Cross-talk between estrogen receptor and epidermal growth factor receptor in head and neck squamous cell carcinoma. *Clin. Cancer Res.* 15:6529-6540, 2009.

[91] Massarweh S., Schiff R.: Resistance to endocrine therapy in breast cancer: exploiting estrogen receptor/growth factor crosstalk. *Endocrin-Related Cancer Suppl.* 13, 1:S15-24, 2006.

[92] Stoner M., Wang F., Wormke M., Nguyen T., Samudio I., Vyhlidal C., Marme D., Finkenzeller G., Safe S.: Inhibition of vascular endothelial growth factor expression in HEC1A endometrial cancer cells through interactions of estrogen receptor alpha and Sp3 proteins. *J. Biol. Chem.* 275:22769-22779, 2000.
[93] Saceda M., Lippman M. E., Chambon P., Lindsey R. L., Ponglikitmongkol M., Puente M., Martin M. B.: Regulation of the estrogen receptor in MCF-7 cells by estradiol. *Mol. Endocrinol.* 2:1157-1162, 1988.
[94] Schreihofer D. A., Stoler M. H., Shupnik M. A.: Differential expression and regulation of estrogen receptors (ERs) in rat pituitary and cell lines: estrogen decreases ER-(alpha)-protein and estrogen responsiveness. *Endocrinol.* 141:2174-2184, 2000.
[95] Shupnik M. A., Gordon M. S., Chin W. W.: Tissue-specific regulation of rat estrogen receptor mRNAs. *Mol. Endocrinol.* 3:660-665, 1989.
[96] Suba Z.: Estrogen deficiency as cancer risk factor. Chapter 5. pp. 85-105. in: Estrogen versus Cancer. Nova Science Publishers Inc, New York 2009.
[97] Liehr J. G.: Is estradiol a genotoxic and mutagenic carcinogen? *Endocrine Rev.* 21:40-54, 2000.
[98] Santen R. J., Martel J., Hoagland M., Naftolin F., Roa L., Harada N., Hafer L., Zaino R., Santner S. J.: Stromal spindle cells contain aromatase in human breast-tumors. *J. Clin. Endocrin. Metab.* 79:627-632, 1994.
[99] Suzuki T., Miki Y., Akahira J. I., Moriya T., Ohuchi N., Sasano H.: Review: Aromatase in human breast carcinoma as a key regulator of intratumoral sex steroid concentrations. *Endocrine J.* 55:455-463, 2008.
[100] Sasano H., Miki Y., Nagasaki S., Suzuki T.: In situ estrogen production and its regulation in human breast carcinoma: From endocrinology to intracrinology. *Pathology International* 59:777-789, 2009.
[101] Hayes D. F.: Tamoxifen: Dr. Jekyll and Mr. Hyde? *J. Natl. Cancer Inst.* 96:895-897, 2004.
[102] Jiang J., Sarwar N., Peston D., Kulinskaya E., Shousha S. Coombes R. C.. Ali S.: Phosporylation of estrogen receptor-alpha at Ser167 is indicative of longer disease-free and overall survival in breast cancer patients. *Clin. Cancer Res.* 13:5769-5776, 2007.
[103] Osborne C. K.: Tamoxifen in the treatment of breast cancer. *N. Engl. J. Med.* 339:1609-1618, 1998.
[104] Early Breast Cancer Trialist's Collaborative Group: Tamoxifen for early breast cancer: an overview of the randomized trials. *Lancet* 351:1451-1467, 1998.
[105] McGuire W. L.: Estrogen receptors in human breast cancer. *J. Clin. Invest.* 52:73-77, 1973.
[106] Bast R. C. Jr., Ravdin P., Hayes D. F., Bates S., Fritsche H. Jr., Jessup J. M., Kemeny N., Locker G. Y., Mennel R. G., Somerfield M. R.: Update of recommendations for the use of tumor markers in breast and colorectal cancer: clinical practice guidelines of the American Society of Clinical Oncology. *J. Clin. Oncol.* 19:1865-1878, 2001.
[107] Gustaffson J. A.: Therapeutic potential of selective estrogen receptor modulators. *Curr. Opin. Chem. Biol.* 2:508-511, 1998.
[108] MacGregor J. I., Jordan V. C.: Basic guide to the mechanisms of antiestrogen action. *Pharmacol. Rev.* 50:151-196, 1998.

[109] McDonald C. C., Alexander F. E., Whyte B. W., Forrest A. P., Stewart H. J.: Cardiac and vascular morbidity in women receiving adjuvant tamoxifen for breast cancer in a randomized trial. The Scottish Cancer Trials Breast Group. *B. M. J.* 311:977-980, 1995.

[110] Stoica A., Saceda M., Doraiswamy V. L., Coleman C., Martin M. B.: Regulation of estrogen receptor-alpha gene expression by epidermal growth factor. *J. Endocrinol.* 165:371-378, 2000.

[111] Parvez S., Tabassum H., Banerjee B. D., Raisuddin S.: Taurine prevents tamoxifen induced mitochondrial oxidative damage in mice. *Basic Clin. Pharmacol. Toxicol.* 102:382-387, 2008.

[112] Ellis M. J., Gao F., Dehdashti F., Jeffe D. B., Marcom P. K., Carey L. A., Dickler M. N., Silverman P., Fleming G. F., Kommareddy A., Jamalabadi-Majidi S., Crowder R., Siegel B. A.: Lower-dose versus high dose oral estradiol therapy of hormone receptor-positive, aromatase inhibitor-resistant advanced breast cancer: A phase 2 randomized study. *J. A. M. A.* 302:774-780, 2009.

In: Estrogen Prevention for Breast Cancer
Editor: Zsuzsanna Suba

ISBN: 978-1-62417-378-3

Chapter VIII

Evolution of Estrogen Action in Breast Cancer: From Culprit to Killer

*Mark B. Leick and V. Craig Jordan**
Georgetown Lombardi Comprehensive Cancer Center, Washington DC, US

Abstract

The rise of tamoxifen as the first targeted therapy for breast cancer that started in 1972 and the subsequent decades of research into hormonal therapy have saved the lives of hundreds of thousands of women. Continuing mechanistic studies elucidated the ability of tamoxifen to act as a selective estrogen receptor modulator (SERM), maintaining or building bone density and lowering circulating cholesterol, while reducing the risk of cancer in the breast. This pharmacologic research gave rise to raloxifene and a whole new drug group, the SERMs. However, through the study of antihormone resistance a surprise was in store with the discovery of a new biology of physiologic estrogen action. After years of adapting to an estrogen deficient environment, due to estrogen deprivation or antiestrogen treatment, breast cancer cells reconfigure their response to the former trophic factor, estrogen, into a potent apoptotic trigger. Estrogen can be used to treat antihormone resistant metastatic breast cancer, but more importantly, the finding of the Women's Health Initiative (WHI) that conjugated equine estrogen alone can reduce mortality by a significant decrease in total cancer and can be explained by the new apoptotic biology of estrogen.

Introduction

The story of the discovery of synthetic estrogens in the 1930s that replicate the action of the natural steroids estradiol and estrone in a woman's body was a major triumph in

* Correspondence to: V. Craig Jordan, OBE, DSc, PhD, FMed Sci, Scientific Director, Georgetown Lombardi Comprehensive Cancer Center, 3970 Reservoir Rd., N. W., Washington, D. C. 20057, US.

elucidating the structure function relationships of an unknown target [1-3]. Estrogen action is very specific in its target sites around the body. When the uterus grows, the quiescent cells of the vagina go through replication and cornification causing an estrogen spike that is essential for ovulation; estrogen is implicated in the growth of breast cancer. By the 1950's the question was how?

The technology to prepare high specific activity tritiated estrogens was the key to all future advances. The discovery of the potent synthetic estrogen diethylstilbestrol (DES) [1] (Figure 1) and the knowledge that potent estrogenic activity could be retained by hydrogenation of the central stilbene double bond, allowed tritiation to be performed and the resulting [^{3}H] hexestrol (Figure 1) used as a tool *in vivo*. The first studies by Glascock and Hoekstra [4] demonstrated specific binding in the estrogen target tissues of sheep and goats. Indeed, subsequent studies were to demonstrate why some breast tumors responded to endocrine ablation in post-menopausal women. Only those patients whose breast tumor accumulated [^{3}H]hexestrol following systemic administration responded to endocrine ablation [5]. The subsequent work of Jensen and Jacobson [6], tritiating 17β estradiol (Figure 1) and using this to beautifully describe the selective binding and retention of [^{3}H] estradiol in the target tissues (uterus, vagina, and pituitary gland) of the immature female rat, really opened the door to all subsequent advances in research on estrogen action. However, it was the finding by Toft and Gorski [7] that the estrogen receptor (ER) was an extractable protein from estrogen target tissues, and indeed the protein could be liganded with [^{3}H]estradiol *in vitro* after extraction from target tissues was an important strategic advance in endocrinology [8]. The ER (and subsequently the whole family of steroid hormone receptors) was unique and not membrane bound like all other pharmacological targets known to exist at that time. Estrogen receptors were present in some breast tumors and not others; the ones with ER were estrogen dependent and could be treated with antiestrogen strategies (i.e. nonsteroidal antiestrogens or aromatase inhibitors).

This short introduction of early laboratory discoveries provides the background and basis for all subsequent laboratory and clinical advances in our knowledge of how to treat and prevent breast cancer through the application of principles defined in the laboratory. We will describe these major advances in medicine but we will also emphasize the new biology of estrogen action that has emerged from the dissection of the evolution of antihormone resistance to antihormone therapy [9]. Here we will describe the changing fashions in breast cancer treatment but emphasize the paradox that occurred right at the beginning of a new era of chemical therapy to treat cancer. Professor Paul Ehrlich was the pioneer in the 19th century who first created a chemical therapy to treat a fatal disease syphilis [10]. In contrast, no advances in cancer therapy were to occur until the 1940's, strangely enough with an application of synthetic estrogen for breast cancer treatment.

The first successful chemical therapy for the treatment of any cancer was the use of high-dose synthetic estrogen for the treatment of metastatic breast cancer [11]. Response rates for patients who were more than a decade beyond menopause were about 30%. Importantly, treatment near menopause was ineffective, and therefore, tumor responsiveness was related to the duration of estrogen deprivation. In 1970, Alexander Haddow commented that "the extraordinary extent of tumor regression observed in perhaps 1% of postmenopausal cases [with estrogen] has always been regarded as of major theoretical importance, and it is a matter for some disappointment that so much of the underlying mechanisms continues to elude us" [12]. High dose estrogen therapy using DES remained the standard of care for the treatment of metastatic breast cancer in postmenopausal women for 30 years (1950s to late 1970s in the United States). However, triphenylethylene-based estrogens evolved into nonsteroidal anti-estrogens [13], where the initial interest focused on their potential as postcoital antifertility agents. This application failed, and the compounds were subsequently reinvented as antiestrogens targeted to ER for the treatment of all stages of breast cancer [14, 15].

Evolution of Fashions in Breast Cancer Treatment and Prevention

The strategy of targeting ER and using long-term adjuvant tamoxifen therapy for breast cancer treatment [14] has increased 15-year survival rates [16, 17] and contributed significantly to the national reduction in breast cancer mortality [18]. From 1975 to 1990, breast cancer mortality rates held roughly steady, but from 1990 to 2000, they declined by 19.6%. It is estimated that about two-thirds of this reduction is because of therapy and one-third is because of mammography screening. Specifically, in ER-positive tumors, 5 years of tamoxifen therapy was estimated to have reduced the hazard of breast cancer mortality by 37%. Tamoxifen (Figure 1) remains the antihormone treatment of choice for the adjuvant treatment of breast cancer in premenopausal patients, despite the development of the aromatase inhibitors (AIs) for the adjuvant treatment of postmenopausal patients with ER-positive breast cancer.

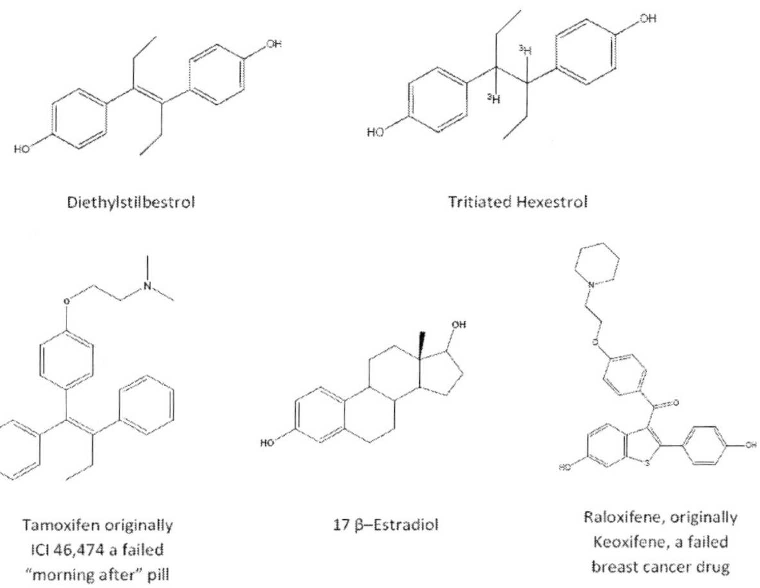

Figure 1. A comparison of the structures of the potent steroidal and nonsteroidal estrogens 17β-estradiol, diethylstilbestrol (DES), [^{3}H] hexestrol and the non-steroidal antiestrogens (now called SERMs) tamoxifen and raloxifene. Tamoxifen and raloxifene are both approved in the US for the reduction of risk for breast cancer in high risk pre and postmenopausal women or postmenopausal women alone respectively.

The AIs provide a modest, but significant, improvement in disease-free survival for patients and a significant decrease in the incidence of both endometrial cancer and thromboembolism associated with tamoxifen therapy in postmenopausal women [19]. Nevertheless, tamoxifen remains an important and cheap lifesaving drug, available in countries without a sophisticated healthcare infrastructure.

Subsequently, the nonsteroidal antiestrogens would again evolve and be reinvented as selective ER modulators (SERMs) [20]. This new drug class exploited the observations that they blocked breast cancer development and growth as antiestrogens but lowered circulating cholesterol and maintained bone density as estrogens. This finding led to the idea that the treatment and prevention of osteoporosis would simultaneously prevent breast cancer [13, 21]. Raloxifene (Figure 1) is the first SERM of the class used to prevent both osteoporosis and breast cancer [22, 23].

Selective ER Modulation: Translation from the Laboratory to Clinical Practice

The original work to investigate the target site pharmacology of tamoxifen in the laboratory provide a database with which to predict clinical outcomes and safety for future chemoprevention trials. Historically in the 1960's there was general interest in the chance finding that nonsteroidal antiestrogens lowered circulating cholesterol. Unfortunately severe toxicological findings were an issue for some compounds because of their ability to increase the level of circulatory desmosterol, which was associated with cataract formation. This toxicity made a search for safer antiestrogens imperative [15]. The discovery of ICI 46,474, the pure trans isomer of the substituted triphenylethylene that was to become tamoxifen, was notable because there was a low conversion to desmosterol though circulating cholesterol was lowered profoundly in rats [24]. Indeed the first patent application for tamoxifen in the U.K. stated [15] in 1965.

> "The alkene derivatives of the invention are useful for the modification of the endocrine status in man and animals and they may be useful for the control of hormone-dependent tumors or for the management of the sexual cycle and aberrations thereof. They also have useful hypocholesterolaemic activity".

However, the patent was denied in the US and the statements concerning breast cancer had to be removed initially as the claim was considered to be "fantastic" and without experimental evidence. The patent for tamoxifen in the United States was finally awarded in 1986 just at the time that the National Cancer Institute recommended adjuvant tamoxifen as the standard of care for patients with ER positive breast cancer [25].

During the 1980s the Wisconsin Tamoxifen study followed up the question of tamoxifen treatment lowering circulating cholesterol in postmenopausal patients [26, 27] and noted a decrease in low density lipoprotein cholesterol but no effect on high density lipoprotein cholesterol. There was certainly some initial enthusiasm that there would be a significant decrease in coronary heart disease but despite some encouraging reports [28-30] no consistent decrease in coronary events has been noted in the Oxford Overview Analysis [Early Breast Cancer Trialists Collaborative Group, [16, 17]] for tamoxifen treatment.

Tamoxifen maintains bone density in ovariectomized rats [21, 31, 32] and this counterintuitive laboratory result for an "antiestrogen" formed the scientific basis for the Wisconsin Tamoxifen Study. The clinical study was a placebo controlled double blind trial to establish the actions of 2 years tamoxifen on bone density in post-menopausal patients with node negative breast cancer (at the time of recruitment, these patients were several years post diagnosis and surgery and no adjuvant treatment was the standard of care). Tamoxifen significantly improved bone density compared to placebo treatment [33].

Thus tamoxifen was estrogen-like, lowering circulating cholesterol and estrogen-like, maintaining bone density so tamoxifen might provide benefit for women enrolled in a chemoprevention trial. The anticancer actions of tamoxifen were well established and supported by the inhibition of mammary carcinogenesis in rat [34, 35] and mouse [36] models. But an increase in the incidence in endometrial cancer was a predictable concern, based on earlier work [37, 38] before major clinical trials of chemoprevention in breast cancer started. Also the finding that tamoxifen was a hepatocarcinogen in specific rat strains [39] was of significance toxicologically for safety reasons in any chemopreventive trials , however, it is fair to say that no evidence either at that time[40, 41] or subsequently has demonstrated hepatocarcinogenesis in humans with tamoxifen. The first pilot chemoprevention study was initiated by Trevor Powles at the Royal Marsden Hospital in the early 1980's [42]. This study grew over the years of accrual and interestingly showed benefit at 20 years for those women taking tamoxifen for 8 years following recruitment [43]. However, the pivotal chemoprevention study was the Fisher P-1 study (Figure 2) conducted by the National Surgical Advent Breast and Bowel Project (NSABP) [44]. This landmark study was an adequately powered prospective, placebo controlled trial primarily used by the Food and Drug Administration as evidence to approve tamoxifen for the reduction of risk of breast cancer in pre and post-menopausal women at high risk for the disease.

There are significant benefits for women at risk for breast cancer nested within the results of the P-1 prevention trial during treatment with tamoxifen. There were fewer fractures but this was not significant overall. Tamoxifen reduces ER positive invasive breast cancer incidence by 50% and the same is true for ductal carcinoma in situ (DCIS) [44]. Benefits in breast chemoprevention last for years following the cessation of treatment [45] and this has been confirmed by others [46]. This is clearly a consistent long term "antitumor action" of tamoxifen imprinted following therapy as noted by the sustained antitumor effect of tamoxifen following adjuvant treatment [16, 17]. We will comment further on the new concept of "imprinting" later in this paper as it pertains to the finding, the estrogen replacement therapy (ERT) can sustain a decrease in breast cancer incidence long after treatment stops [47].

Despite extensive testing, tamoxifen is seen as presenting the well woman with significant risks such as endometrial cancer and blood clots (it must be stressed that this is observed only in postmenopausal women) [44] (Figure 3). There is also the nagging concern about rat hepatocarcinoma. Tamoxifen has a human carcinogen black box designation in the US With all these uncertainties, clearly another strategy for chemoprevention was necessary for an appropriate science based advance in public health. This was obvious [13] even before the NSABP trial had been launched in the early 1990's [44]but tamoxifen was the only medicine available with sufficient clinical trials experience to move forward into chemoprevention. Nevertheless, the recognition of SERMs in the laboratory [13] also catalyzed a change in the development of another nonsteroidal antiestrogen keoxifene (Figure 1). Keoxifene was initially investigated in the 1980s as a competitor for tamoxifen as a breast cancer drug but which failed to advance in development as it failed in clinical trial [48]. Surprisingly, keoxifene also maintained bone density in rats similar to tamoxifen but was significantly less uterotrophic than tamoxifen [21]. This would later translate to a reduced risk of endometrial cancer in all subsequent clinical trials. The name was changed from keoxifene to raloxifene (Figure 1). Keoxifene prevented mammary cancer in rats but because of poor pharmacokinetics and rapid excretion keoxifene does not have the sustained actions of tamoxifen [34].

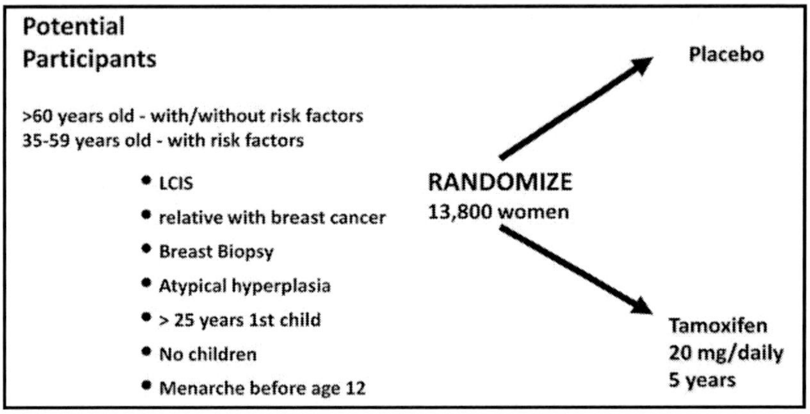

Figure 2. The risk requirements for recruitment to the National Surgical Breast and Bowel Project (NSABP)/National Cancer Institute (NCI) study P-1 to determine the worth of tamoxifen for preventing breast cancer in high risk pre and postmenopausal women [44].

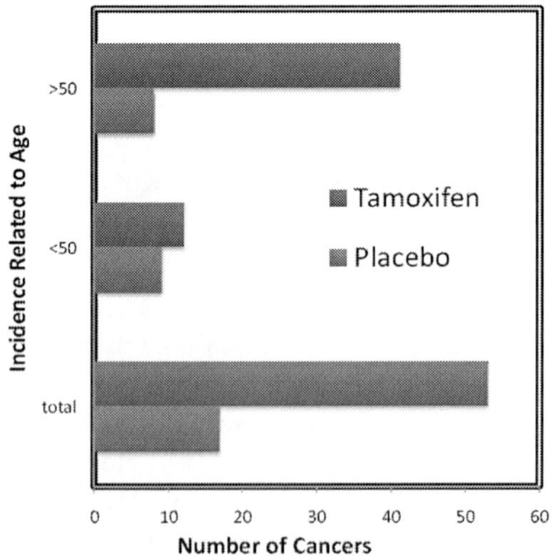

Figure 3. The total and age related incidence of endometrial cancer in the NSABP/NCI P-1 chemoprevention trial [45]. Premenopausal women have no increased risk of developing endometrial cancer during or following 5 years of tamoxifen treatment.

Continuous therapy was necessary. Thus the scene was set for a move away from a broad therapeutic strategy with tamoxifen administered to high risk populations where a few ER positive invasive breast cancers can be prevented but the majority of women are exposed to side effects with no benefit to balance the risks. In response, a "roadmap" was created based on laboratory science and the emerging clinical trial data that would significantly advance women's health.

A Roadmap to Use SERMS to Prevent Multiple Diseases in Women

A plan to prevent breast cancer as a public health initiative was initially described at the First International Chemoprevention meeting in New York in 1987 [49]. It is reasonable simply to state the proposal, published from the 1987 meeting [49] "*The majority of breast cancer occurs unexpectedly and from unknown origin. Great efforts are being focused on the identification of a population of high-risk women to test "chemopreventive" agents. But, are resources being used less than optimally? An alternative would be to seize on the developing clues provided by an extensive clinical investigation of available antiestrogens. Could analogues be developed to treat osteoporosis or even retard the development of atherosclerosis? If this proved to be true, then a majority of women in general would be treated for these conditions as soon as menopause occurred. Should the agent also retain anti-breast tumor actions, then it might be expected to act as a chemosuppressive on all developing breast cancers if these have an evolution from hormone-dependent disease to hormone-independent disease. A bold commitment to drug discovery and clinical pharmacology will potentially place us in a key position to prevent the development of breast cancer by the end of this century [49]"*. The vision of the concept was refined and focused by 1990 [13]. "*We have obtained valuable clinical information about this group of drugs that can be applied in other disease states. Research does not travel in straight lines and observations in one field of science often become major discoveries in another. Important clues have been garnered about the effects of tamoxifen on bone and lipids, so apparently, derivatives could find targeted applications to retard osteoporosis or atherosclerosis. The ubiquitous application of novel compounds to prevent diseases associated with the progressive changes after menopause may, as a side effect, significantly retard the development of breast cancer. The target population would be postmenopausal women in general, thereby avoiding the requirement to select a high-risk group to prevent breast cancer.*" This concept is exactly what has been translated to clinical practice [22, 50]: use a SERM (raloxifene) to treat osteoporosis and reduce the incidence of breast cancer as a beneficial side effect [22, 50, 51].

Raloxifene in Clinical Practice

Raloxifene is the pioneering SERM approved for the prevention of osteoporosis around the world. The pivotal registration trial was the Multiple Outcomes of Raloxifene Evaluation

(MORE) trial. Raloxifene reduced spine fractures by 50% compared to placebo [51]. A separate analysis of breast cancer incidence demonstrated a 76% decrease in the incidence of invasive positive breast cancer (Figure 4) over the 3 year evaluation. There was no increase in endometrial cancer but DCIS remained unaffected [22].

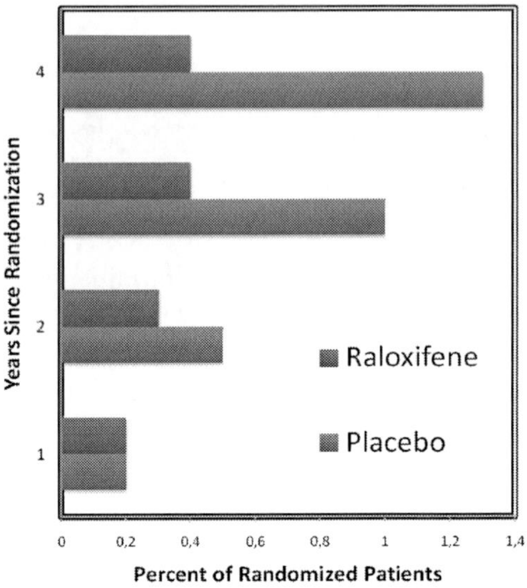

Figure 4. The annual accumulative incidence breast cancers represented as a percent of affected randomized patients in the Multiple Outcomes of Raloxifene Evaluation (MORE) that randomized women with an increased risk for osteoporotic fractures to placebo (2576 women) or raloxifene (5129 women) [22].

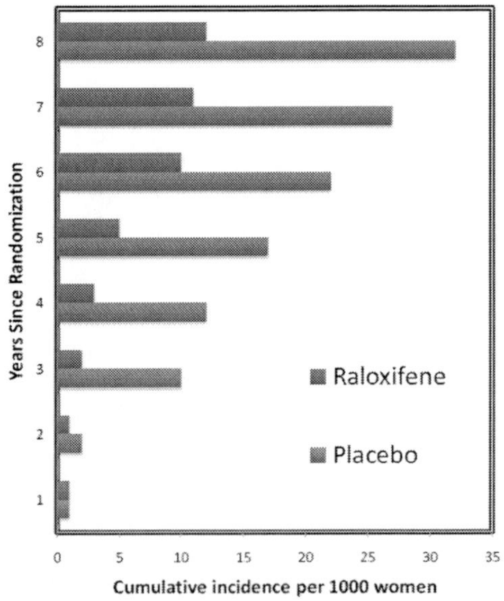

Figure 5. The cumulative incidence of invasive breast cancer for the combined MORE and Continuing Outcomes Relevant to Evista (CORE) studies. Shown are patients at high risk for osteoporotic fractures receiving either placebo or raloxifene (60mg daily) [50].

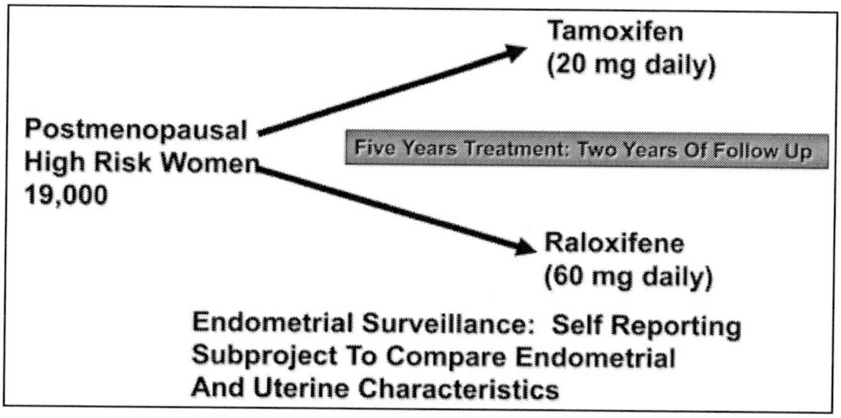

Figure 6. The design of the Study of Tamoxifen and Raloxifene (STAR). The STAR trial for postmenopausal women at elevated risk for breast cancer had fewer serious side effects when taking raloxifene but a similar reduction in the incidence of breast cancer [23]. However, after stopping the SERM treatment, the antitumor action of raloxifene was not maintained [101] so continuous treatment with raloxifene is recommended (as this is the approval for the treatment and prevention of osteoporosis).

A long running trial, Raloxifene Use for the Heart (RUTH), to examine whether coronary heart events could be reduced in high risk populations, did not show benefit for raloxifene [52]. Looked at another way, it showed little harm, but coronary heart disease (CHD) in a high risk population was unaffected.

The use of estrogen-like medicines to treat and prevent osteoporosis in the postmenopausal woman demands long term therapy – perhaps indefinite therapy. The extension trial to MORE was Continuing Outcomes Relevant to Evista (CORE) [50].An evaluation of both breast cancer and endometrial cancer in the CORE trial confirmed a sustained efficacy to prevent the development of breast cancer over the 9 years of raloxifene treatment (Figure 5) and this effect was entirely expressed in the prevention of ER positive disease with no effect on the development of ER negative disease.

Not surprisingly, the promising data from the MORE trial [22] would propel raloxifene into a head to head study of tamoxifen and raloxifene (STAR) in high risk postmenopausal women (Figure 6). The STAR trial teaches several important lessons. However the dramatic decrease in invasive breast cancer noted in the MORE trial (raloxifene reducing the risk of ER positive breast cancer by 90% - and a 76% reduction of any newly diagnosed invasive breast cancer) [22] was not noted in STAR with raloxifene. There was no difference between the incidence of breast cancer during treatment with tamoxifen or raloxifene [23] notwithstanding the presumed 50% decrease based on the results from the P-1 trial [44, 45]. Raloxifene had a very low proliferative effect on the uterine epithelium when compared with tamoxifen and this translated to fewer hysterectomies in the raloxifene treated women [23]. Additionally there were fewer thrombotic events with raloxifene and fewer operations for cataracts (see earlier concerns with the triphenylethylene based nonsteroidal antiestrogens [15]). Overall raloxifene seems to be equivalent to tamoxifen as a chemopreventive for invasive breast cancer but raloxifene is less effective than tamoxifen at controlling the development of DCIS. Nevertheless, raloxifene confers greater safety.

However, the importance of long term follow up for clinical trials is illustrated by STAR. A recent evaluation of the STAR trial 3 years after stopping the 5 years of treatment showed that although tamoxifen retained its "imprinting" as an antitumor agent raloxifene did not. Raloxifene was only 78% as effective at reducing primary breast cancer incidence as tamoxifen. These clinical data [23] reflect the superiority of tamoxifen in preclinical studies [34] and based on the raloxifene extension study, raloxifene [50] may need to be given indefinitely to prevent both osteoporosis and breast cancer.

Summary of SERMs

The central principle for the successful treatment or prevention of breast cancer with any antihormone is the application of the strategy of long term therapy. By definition, breast cancer that is exposed to such a continuous strategy will be selected for a growth advantage and disease will become resistant to treatment and progress. To presage this inevitable course for cancer, laboratory studies were initiated in the 1980's to address the mechanisms of SERM resistance by developing clinically relevant models using available breast cancer cell lines. Similar studies also addressed the acquired resistance of breast cancer to estrogen deprivation in anticipation of the success of aromatase inhibitors applied to adjuvant antihormone therapy in postmenopausal patients. However, a surprise was in store with the discovery of the evolution of antihormone resistance in response to sustained antihormone therapy.

The Evolution of Acquired Resistance to Antihormonal Therapies

Twenty years ago, we took a long-term view by creating a whole range of breast and endometrial cancer models resistant to tamoxifen and raloxifene [53-57]. Our goal was to anticipate the clinical development of drug resistance and to understand mechanisms so that second-line therapies could be deployed rationally. The models were developed naturally by first establishing estrogen stimulated tumor growth in athymic mice followed by long-term SERM treatment to identify SERM-resistant tumors. All our models were retransplanted into subsequent generations of mice so that the impact of long-term SERM therapy could be evaluated in hormone-responsive breast and endometrial cancer. SERM resistance is unique because both breast and endometrial tumors grow in response to either SERMs or estrogen. No estrogen (mimicking aromatase inhibitor treatment) or the use of a pure antiestrogen (ICI 164,384 [58] or fulvestrant [59, 60]) prevent SERM resistant tumor growth. This is why aromatase inhibitors or fulvestrant are effective second-line therapies after tamoxifen failure [61, 62].

However, the early models of SERM resistance did not reflect the majority of clinical experience. The natural laboratory models developed during a year of therapy [53, 63] and therefore reflected drug resistance in patients with metastatic breast cancer who are only treated successfully for 1 year. We took the strategic decision to determine what would occur if breast tumors were retransplanted into successive generations of tamoxifen stimulated mice for 5 years or more (i.e., to replicated the actual clinical conditions employed during long-term adjuvant therapy). Remarkably, drug resistance evolves and the survival signaling pathway in tamoxifen resistant tumors becomes reorganized so that instead of estrogen being a survival signal, physiologic estrogen now inhibits tumor growth. This discovery [55, 64] provided an invaluable insight into the evolution of drug resistance to SERMs and prompted the reclassification of the process through phase I (SERM/estrogen stimulated growth) and phase II (SERM stimulated growth estrogen inhibited growth) (Figure 7).

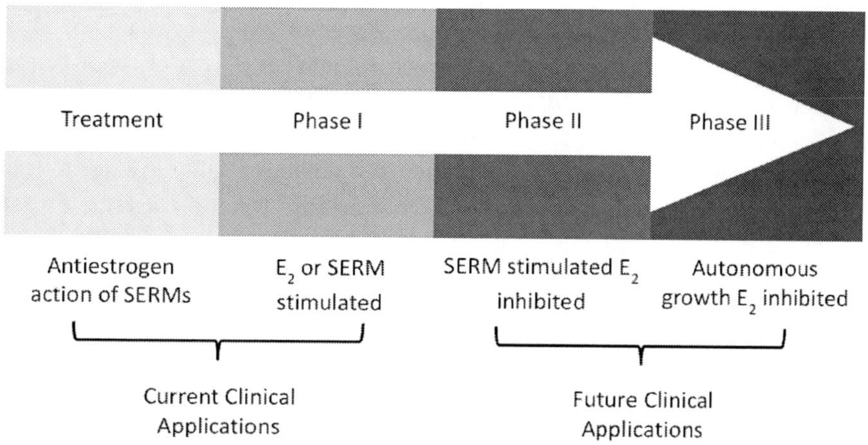

Figure 7. Evolution of drug resistance to selective estrogen receptor modulations (SERMs). Acquired resistance occurs during long-term treatment with a SERM and is evidenced by SERM-stimulated breast tumor growth. Tumors also continue to exploit estrogen for growth when the SERM is stopped, so a dual signal transduction process develops. The aromatase inhibitors prevent tumor growth in SERM-resistant disease and fulvestrant that destroys the estrogen receptor (ER) is also effective. This phase of drug resistance is referred to as phase I resistance. Continued exposure to a SERM results in continued SERM-stimulated growth, but eventually autonomous growth occurs that is unresponsive to fulvestrant or aromatase inhibitors. The event that distinguishes phase I from phase II acquired resistance is a remarkable switching mechanism that now causes apoptosis, rather than growth, with physiologic levels of estrogen. These distinct phases of laboratory-drug resistance [55, 67] have their clinical parallels and this new knowledge is being integrated into the treatment plan.

The apoptotic action of physiological estrogen to cause dramatic tumor regression of long-term tamoxifen-resistant ER-positive breast cancers grown in athymic mice [55, 64] was subsequently extended to long-term raloxifene resistance [65, 66] and ER-positive breast cancer cells maintained in an estrogen-deprived environment for prolonged periods [67-71]. Most importantly, the apoptotic results observed with estrogen-deprived cells were noted both in vitro and in vivo by inoculation into athymic mice [67].

Molecular Mechanisms of the Apoptotic Action of Estrogens

The underlying mechanism behind tumor regression in response to high dose estrogen in post menopausal women that eluded Alexander Haddow [12] is now becoming clear. It is well known that estrogen has inherent carcinogenic properties via oxidative metabolites that covalently bind to DNA and proteins and oxidative damage [72] as well as through ER signaling pathways [73] including transcriptional alteration of nuclear and mitochondrial encoded genes and second messenger systems like the MAPK family and cAMP-responsive genes [72]. Conveniently, the logical pharmacological intervention at this level (SERMs and aromatase inhibitors) provides a viable treatment strategy [74]. However, the paradoxical results of the Women's Health Initiative (WHI) ,a double-blind, placebo-controlled randomized trial in which 10,739 postmenopausal women with prior hysterectomy (ages 50-79) were treated with estrogen replacement therapy (ERT), which showed a decrease in invasive breast cancer which was sustained for 5 years after ERT was stopped, again raised the possibility of estrogen as a viable therapy for, rather than driver of, breast cancer [47, 75]. New evidence shows that physiologic estrogen may actually induce apoptosis by linking the estrogen receptor to apoptotic triggers [76].

Estrogen therapy in the 1940s was the first chemical therapy to treat any cancer successfully [11] and became the standard of care to treat metastatic breast cancer in postmenopausal patients until the introduction of tamoxifen which became the standard of care for the next 20 years. In a comparison of the synthetic estrogen DES to tamoxifen, the two showed similar responses initially with more side effects in the DES group [77], though a follow-up analysis showed a significant improvement in survival with DES with a 5 year survival of 35% vs. 16% (p=.039) [78]. With the rise of tamoxifen, much of the research into the antitumor activity of estrogen analogs stalled save for at least one animal model which found similar antitumor responses to high dose estrogen in tumors transplanted into nude mice [79, 80].

The first molecular evidence that estrogen at physiologic concentrations could indeed activate apoptosis demonstrated that cell death could occur through the extrinsic pathway through induction of Fas [81] or Fas ligand [70] with concomitant suppression of antiapoptotic and prosurvival signals HER2/neu and NF-kappaB [81]. Crucially, it was shown in cell culture and animal models that physiologic concentrations of estradiol could also induce apoptosis [82, 83].

Mechanistic studies, [70, 81] using unique laboratory models, demonstrate that the antihormone resistant cells have reconfigured the ER signal transduction pathway so despite the fact that the ER still regulates the appropriate estrogen-regulated genes (including pS_2 and *myc)*[84] there is a profound effect of estrogen to activate the fas (death) receptor system or to alternatively have a direct effect on mitochondrial function via the bcl2 system [81, 85]. Later studies further revealed that estrogen could induce the alternative intrinsic mitochondrial apoptotic pathway with increased cytochrome c release [67].

Recent global gene expression analysis [86] in cells susceptible to estrogen induced apoptosis shows that estrogen signaling, endoplasmic reticulum stress, and inflammatory response genes are upregulated compared to controls. Estrogen signaling is suppressed by metabolically reducing intracellular estradiol concentrations (increased CYP1B1 and HDS17B11) and upregulating genes that antagonize ERα activity (SETD7, FHL2,Snail 1, COUP-TF1, TRα, AR, INHBA, and SMAD3) or repressing genes that promote ERα activity (AREG, PIK3CB, and CAV1). endoplasmic reticulum stress was indicated by a deficiency in up-regulating genes involved in initiating a UPR (GRP78, XBP1, and S1P), protein folding (GRP78, PDIA6, and UGGT1), and degradation of malfolded proteins (HERP1 and DERL1), which would lead to accumulation of unfolded/misfolded proteins. Meanwhile, expression profiles indicated a widespread inhibition of protein translation (increased p58 IPK and decreased aminoacyl tRNA synthetases, EEF2K, and ERF3A) and fatty acid synthesis (decreased ACLY and SCD), which combined with accumulation of unfolded proteins, would also promote stress and apoptosis. endoplasmic reticulum stress was also indicated by induction of BIM, BAX, and the inflammatory caspase CASP4. Inflammatory stress was indicated by up-regulation of cytokines/cytokine receptors (IL-4R, IL-6R, IL-6ST/gp130, IL-17RD, and LTB), IFN/IFN responsive genes (IFNL1,IFI6, and IFI16), arachidonic acid biosynthetic genes (FADS1 and PLA2G10), and other inflammatory markers (CEBPB, NTN1, and UNC5C). These findings indicate that inflammatory and endoplasmic reticulum stress responses leading to apoptosis are highly interrelated and may cross-talk in part through NF-κB, JNK, and AP-1. Thus, additional stimulation of endoplasmic reticulum stress and inflammatory responses by arachidonic acid interacted with estrogen to superadditively induce apoptosis [86].

Ongoing mechanistic studies demonstrate that the shape of the estrogen-ER complex is critical to trigger apoptosis [87, 88] . Simply stated, if triphenylethylene based estrogen binds to the prepared breast cancer cell ER, but adopts an "antiestrogenic complex" then this delays apoptosis. Coactivators do not bind efficiently to the complex so the shape of the complex and the appropriate delivery of coactivators is part of the trigger for apoptosis. Additionally, use of RNAseq has demonstrated [89] that oxidative stress is a key component of the early events in estrogen induced apoptosis initiated in the mitochondria. Inhibition of estrogen induced apoptosis with 4-hydroxytamoxifen or a cSrc inhibitor blocks the products of reactive oxygen species through a blockade of the AP-1 subunit (cfos, cjun) synthesis.

Thus an understanding of the paradoxical actions of estrogen has emerged that depend on the state of estrogen deprivation of the breast cancer cell. In an estrogen rich environment, the estradiol-ER complex is a survival system promoting tumor growth. In contrast, in an estrogen-deprived environment (treatment with tamoxifen or an aromatase inhibitor) estrogen action is replaced by internal survival signaling based on the selection of cells with enhanced growth factor receptors. The growth factor receptors [90] initiate cascades that phosphorylate either unoccupied ER or ER liganded by SERMs. This model would also explain the earlier observations why high-dose estrogen therapy was only effective as a treatment for breast cancer in woman many years after menopause [12]. Natural estrogen deprivation had occurred. The process is accelerated and enhanced, however, in patients treated long-term with SERMs or aromatase inhibitors so that only low doses of estrogen are necessary to cause experimental tumors to regress.

Clinical Significance of Estrogen Induced Apoptosis

There is now very strong clinical evidence that estrogen may work against active disease. A very encouraging study by Lønning et. al. [91] of high dose DES in the setting of metastatic breast cancer following exhaustive antihormone therapy (tamoxifen, aromatase inhibitors, etc.) resulted in 4 of 32 patients having complete responses and another patient having no recurrence of her disease six years after stopping DES [91, 92]. A later clinical trial by Ellis et. al. [93] found similar efficacy for both low (6mg/day) and high (30mg/day) dose estradiol in patients who had progressed on aromatase inhibitor therapy achieving clinical benefit rates of 28% and 29% respectively.

Some of the strongest clinical evidence to support the hypothesis that physiologic estrogen is apoptotic comes from the results of the WHI trial indicating that estrogen may have a role in reducing the incidence of breast cancer and a sustained reduction in breast cancer incidence even after cessation of therapy for a median of 4.7 years [47]. Initial analysis of the WHI trial at a mean follow-up of 7.1 years found that while there was an increase in mammograms requiring follow-up in the treatment group the incidence of invasive breast cancer was not increased compared to placebo, hazard ratio 0.8 (95% CI 0.62-1.04, p=.09) [94]. Later, LaCroix et. al. [47] followed up on the same WHI estrogen trial with a mean follow-up time of 10.7 years and found that conjugated equine estrogen use for a mean of 5.9 years lead to a reduced breast cancer incidence compared to control (0.27% vs. 0.35% respectively, HR 0.77; 95% CI, 0.62-0.95) that remained even after therapy was stopped with no difference between the intervention and post intervention phases [75]. At a median follow-up time of 11.8 years Anderson et. al. [75] found that breast cancer risk reduction with estrogen was primarily in women without benign breast disease or a family history, and that fewer women in the estrogen group died from breast cancer (HR 0.37 p=.03) or any cause (HR 0.62, p=.04) after a breast cancer diagnosis compared to control. However, the authors urged caution with interpretation of the findings due to the fact that the risk reduction was not seen in those with a first degree relative with breast cancer [75], highlighting the need for careful subgroup selection. The data also revealed that reduction of breast cancer risk may be related to an increased delay (>5 years) in initiation of ERT [95], further buttressing the notion that the estrogen receptor undergoes remodeling into an apoptotic trigger under conditions of prolonged estrogen deprivation.

Several older studies show similar results consistent with the idea that estrogen is playing a protective role in carefully selected women. A large prospective cohort study of 422,373 postmenopausal women showed that use of ERT was associated with a significantly decreased risk of fatal breast cancer (RR = 0.84) after 9 years of follow-up and 1,469 breast cancer deaths [96].

A variety of data supports the notion that estrogen alone may be more promising than combination with progestin. A trial with estrogen plus progestin rather than estrogen alone in 16,608 postmenopausal women with no prior hysterectomy resulted in an increase in invasive breast cancer (HR 1.25, p=.004) with an increased likelihood of being node positive (HR 1.78, p = .03) [97]. The distinction was seen in other areas as well. The difference in incidence in lung cancer in the WHI for conjugated equine estrogen alone compared to placebo at a mean follow up of 7.9 years was not significant with 0.15% vs. 0.13% respectively (HR 1.17, 95% CI: 0.81 to 1.69, p=0.39), nor was there a difference in number, stage, grade, or mortality [98]. Use of estrogen alone was correlated with a significant decrease in mortality from non small cell lung cancer compared to estrogen plus progestin therapy HR 0.48 (95% CI 0.24 to 0.95, p=0.03) [98]. However, in the case of colorectal carcinoma it was estrogen plus progesterone that saw a protective effect though there was no increased incidence for estrogen alone HR 0.56 (95% CI 0.38 to 0.81, p=.003) [98]. In a subgroup analysis, however, it was found that women aged 70-79 had a nearly 2-fold increase risk of colorectal cancer in the conjugated estrogen group [47].

Conclusion

In the quest for knowledge to advance public health, we rely on randomized placebo controlled clinical trials and pertinent laboratory data designed to question Nature. Both sources of knowledge have limitations, but if the answers from our questions are consistent and our controls are sound, public health can advance. The article by Anderson [75] is reassuring to the appropriate women who wish to take CEE at an average of 63 years of age; breast cancer incidence and mortality are decreasing.

Unfortunately, the question being asked of Nature was not when should CEE be started. We will provide scientific evidence in favor of a lengthy estrogen deprived environment prior to CEE based on our knowledge of cancer biology and the new biology estrogen induced apoptosis [99].

Cancer thrives in an environment that promotes growth; breast cancer is no exception. In the transition from an estrogen rich environment to an estrogen poor environment following menopause, cell populations must adapt to austerity. The principle is Darwinian and predicts that populations of cells will perish and new populations will arise adapted to low estrogen levels with growth hypersensitivity to restricted estrogen levels. The further from the menopause, the more profound change to cell survival will become. This principle was illustrated, more than 25 years ago with the ER positive MCF-7 breast cancer cell line upon estrogen withdrawal [100]. The majority of cells die but an estrogen independent ER positive cell population eventually grows, that remain antihormone responsive to inhibit growth. However reintroduction of estrogen does not kill cells but they rapidly re-adapt to estrogen to promote further growth [100]. Only in populations of cells kept under estrogen deprived conditions for years does estrogen inhibit growth [70]. Indeed, some clonal populations are extremely sensitive to estrogen induced apoptosis [67]. The events involved in estrogen induced apoptosis have recently been described [86] and this may account for the significant decrease in some but not all breast cancers with CEE treatment. The key, however, is time of estrogen deprivation and the plasticity of populations to adapt to austerity.

Thus, based on the evidence available, Nature appears to be consistent. It may be that a short period of CEE may be sufficient to control menopausal symptoms in the severe cases and to provide some benefit for the symptomatic few. The fact remains, that the majority of women started CEE at 63 years of age in the WHI and not at the time of the menopause. Perhaps decisions must be made individually to reduce menopausal symptoms for a year now, wait for 5-10 years and reduce the incidence of breast cancer later in life.

Initial studies showed that after cessation of adjuvant tamoxifen a woman's own estrogen would provide an antitumor effect and prolong survival [64] and that subsequently, the tumor is again susceptible to tamoxifen [55]. Further work has found a similar effect for raloxifene and supports a cyclical treatment algorithm consisting of hormonal receptor blockade followed by stimulation upon pathway reconfiguration [65, 66]. Currently, the Study of Letrozole Extension (SOLE) trial is evaluating the use of regular drug holidays with antihormone therapy in an attempt to test the hypothesis that a woman's own estrogen may be sufficient to induce apoptosis in vulnerable cell populations.

It is now clear based on laboratory and clinical studies over the past two decades that estrogen not only is a survival signal for breast cancer cell growth but also, and perhaps surprisingly, an apoptotic trigger for estrogen deprived breast cancer to initiate cell death.

Acknowledgments

This work (VCJ) was supported by the Department of Defense Breast Program under Award number W81XWH-06-1-0590 Center of Excellence; subcontract under the SU2C (AACR) Grant number SU2C-AACR-DT0409; the Susan G Komen For The Cure Foundation under Award number SAC100009; GHUCCTS CTSA (Grant # UL1RR031975) and the Lombardi Comprehensive Cancer Center Support Grant (CCSG) Core Grant NIH P30 CA051008. The content is solely the responsibility of the authors and does not necessarily represent the official views of the National Cancer Institute or the National Institutes of Health. Additionally, the views and opinions of the author(s) do not reflect those of the US Army or the Department of Defense.

References

[1] Dodds E. C., Goldberg L., Lawson W., Robinson R. Oestrogenic activity of certain synthetic compounds. *Nature* 141:247-48, 1938.

[2] Dodds E., Lawson W., Noble R. Biological effects of the synthetic oestrogen substance 4: 4-dihydroxy a beta-diethyl-stilbene. *Lancet* 1:1389-91, 1938.

[3] Robson J., Schönberg A. Oestrous reactions, including mating, produced by triphenyl ethylene. *Nature* 140:196, 1937.

[4] Glascock R., Hoekstra W. Selective accumulation of tritium-labelled hexoestrol by the reproductive organs of immature female goats and sheep. *Biochemical Journal* 72:673-82, 1959.

[5] Folca P., Glascock R., Irvine W. Studies with tritium-labelled hexoestrol in advanced breast cancer. Comparison of tissue accumulation of hexoestrol with response to bilateral adrenalectomy and oophorectomy. *Lancet* 2:796-98, 1961.

[6] Jensen E. V., Jacobson H. I. Basic guides to the mechanism of estrogen action. *Recent Progress in Hormone Research* 18:387-414, 1962.

[7] Toft D., Gorski J. A receptor molecule for estrogens: isolation from the rat uterus and preliminary characterization. *Proceedings of the National Academy of Sciences of the United States of America* 55:1574-81, 1966.

[8] Toft D., Shyamala G, Gorski J. A receptor molecule for estrogens: studies using a cell-free system. *Proceedings of the National Academy of Sciences of the United States of America* 57:1740-43, 1967.

[9] Jordan V. C. Selective estrogen receptor modulation: concept and consequences in cancer. *Cancer Cell* 5:207-13, 2004.

[10] Baumler E. Paul Ehrlich, *Scientist for Life: Holmes and Meier* (New York); 1984.

[11] Haddow A., Watkinson J. M., Paterson E., Koller P. Influence of synthetic oestrogens on advanced malignant disease. *British Medical Journal* 2:393-98, 1944.

[12] Haddow A. David A. Karnofsky memorial lecture. Thoughts on chemical therapy. *Cancer* 26:737-54, 1970.

[13] Lerner L. J., Jordan V. C. Development of antiestrogens and their use in breast cancer: Eighth Cain memorial award lecture. *Cancer Research* 50:4177-89, 1990.

[14] Jordan V. C. Tamoxifen: catalyst for the change to targeted therapy. *European Journal of Cancer* 44:30-38, 2008.

[15] Jordan V. C. Tamoxifen: a most unlikely pioneering medicine. *Nature Reviews Drug Discovery* 2:205-13, 2003.

[16] EBCTCG. Tamoxifen for early breast cancer: an overview of the randomised trials. *Lancet* 351:1451-67, 1998.

[17] EBCTCG. Effects of chemotherapy and hormonal therapy for early breast cancer on recurrence and 15-year survival: an overview of the randomised trials. *Lancet* 365:1687-717, 2005.

[18] Berry D. A., Inoue L., Shen Y., Venier J., Cohen D., Bondy M., et al. Modeling the impact of treatment and screening on US breast cancer mortality: a Bayesian approach. *J. N. C. I. Monographs* 2006:30-36, 2006

[19] Dowsett M., Cuzick J., Ingle J., Coates A., Forbes J., Bliss J, et al. Meta-analysis of breast cancer outcomes in adjuvant trials of aromatase inhibitors versus tamoxifen. *Journal of Clinical Oncology* 28:509-18, 2010.

[20] Jordan V. C. Selective estrogen receptor modulation: A Personal Perspective. *Cancer Research* 61:5683-87, 2001.

[21] Jordan V. C., Phelps E., Lindgren J. U. Effects of anti-estrogens on bone in castrated and intact female rats. *Breast Cancer Research and Treatment* 10:31-35, 1987.

[22] Cummings S. R., Eckert S., Krueger K. A., Grady D., Powles T. J., Cauley J. A., et al. The effect of raloxifene on risk of breast cancer in postmenopausal women : results from the MORE randomized trial. Multiple Outcomes of Raloxifene Evaluation. *The Journal of the American Medical Association* 281:2189-97, 1999.

[23] Vogel V. G., Costantino J. P., Wickerham D. L., Cronin W. M., Cecchini R. S., Atkins J. N., et al. Effects of tamoxifen vs raloxifene on the risk of developing invasive breast cancer and other disease outcomes: the NSABP Study of Tamoxifen and Raloxifene (STAR) P-2 trial. *The Journal of the American Medical Association* 295:2727-41, 2006.

[24] Harper M. J., Walpole A. L. A new derivative of triphenylethylene: effect on implantation and mode of action in rats. *The Journal of the Society for Reproduction and Fertility* 13:101-19, 1967.

[25] Consensus conference. Adjuvant chemotherapy for breast cancer. *The Journal of the American Medical Association* 254:3461-3, 1985.

[26] Love R. R., Newcomb P. A., Wiebe D. A., Surawicz T. S., Jordan V. C., Carbone P. P., et al. Effects of tamoxifen therapy on lipid and lipoprotein levels in postmenopausal patients with node-negative breast cancer. *The Journal of the National Cancer Institute* 82:1327-32, 1990.

[27] Love R. R., Wiebe D. A., Newcomb P. A., Cameron L., Leventhal H., Jordan V. C., et al. Effects of tamoxifen on cardiovascular risk factors in post-menopausal women. *Annals of Internal Medicine* 115:860-4, 1991.

[28] Nordenskjöld B., Rosell J., Rutqvist L. E., Malmström P. O., Bergh J., Bengtsson N. O., et al. Coronary heart disease mortality after 5 years of adjuvant tamoxifen therapy: Results from a randomzed trial. *Journal of the National Cancer Institute* 97:1609-10, 2005.

[29] Hackshaw A., Roughton M., Forsyth S., Monson K., Reczko K., Sainsbury R., et al. Long-term benefits of 5 years of tamoxifen: 10-year follow-up of a large randomized trial in women at least 50 years of ge with early breast cancer. *Journal of Clinical Oncology* 29:1657-63, 2011.

[30] McDonald C. C., Stewart H. J. Fatal myocardial infarction in the Scottish adjuvant tamoxifen trial. The Scottish Breast Cancer Committee. *British Medical Journal* 303:435-37, 1991.

[31] Turner R. T., Wakley G. K., Hannon K. S., Bell N. H. Tamoxifen prevents the skeletal effects of ovarian hormone deficiency in rats. *Journal of Bone and Mineral Research* 2:449-56, 1987.

[32] Turner R. T., Wakley G. K., Hannon K. S., Bell N. H. Tamoxifen inhibits osteoclast-mediated resorption of trabecular bone in ovarian hormone-deficient rats. *Endocrinology* 122:1146-50, 1988.

[33] Love R. R., Mazess R. B., Barden H. S., Epstein S., Newcomb P. A., Jordan V. C., et al. Effects of tamoxifen on bone mineral density in postmenopausal women with breast cancer. *The New England Journal of Medicine* 326:852-6, 1992.

[34] Gottardis M. M., Jordan V. C. Antitumor actions of keoxifene and tamoxifen in the N-nitrosomethylurea-induced rat mammary carcinoma model. *Cancer Research* 47:4020-24, 1987.

[35] Jordan V. C. Effect of tamoxifen (ICI 46,474) on initiation and growth of DMBA-induced rat mammary carcinomata. *European Journal of Cancer* 12:419-24, 1976.

[36] Jordan V. C., Lababidi M. K., Langan-Fahey S. Suppression of mouse mammary tumorigenesis by long-term tamoxifen therapy. *Journal of the National Cancer Institute* 83:492-6, 1991.

[37] Gottardis M. M., Robinson S. P., Satyaswaroop P. G., Jordan V. C. Contrasting actions of tamoxifen on endometrial and breast tumor growth in the athymic mouse. *Cancer Research* 48:812-5, 1988.

[38] Fornander T., Rutqvist L. E., Cedermark B., Glas U., Mattsson A., Silfversward C., et al. Adjuvant tamoxifen in early breast cancer: occurrence of new primary cancers. *Lancet* 1:117-20, 1989.

[39] Greaves P., Goonetilleke R., Nunn G., Topham J., Orton T. Two-year carcinogenicity study of tamoxifen in Alderley Park Wistar-derived rats. *Cancer Research* 53: 3919-24, 1993.

[40] Jordan V. C. What if tamoxifen (ICI 46,474) had been found to produce rat liver tumors in 1973? A personal perspective. *Annals of Oncology* 6:29-34, 1995.

[41] Jordan V. C., Morrow M. Should clinicians be concerned about the carcinogenic potential of tamoxifen? *European Journal of Cancer* 30A:1714-21, 1994.

[42] Powles T. J., Hardy J. R., Ashley S. E., Farrington G. M., Cosgrove D.,

[43] Davey J. B., et al. A pilot trial to evaluate the acute toxicity and feasibility of tamoxifen for prevention of breast cancer. *British Journal of Cancer* 60:126-31, 1989.

[44] Powles T. J., Ashley S., Tidy A., Smith I. E., Dowsett M. Twenty-year follow-up of the Royal Marsden randomized, double-blinded tamoxifen breast cancer prevention trial. *Journal of the National Cancer Institute* 99:283-90, 2007.

[45] Fisher B., Costantino J. P., Wickerham D. L., Redmond C. K., Kavanah M., Cronin W. M., et al. Tamoxifen for prevention of breast cancer: report of the National

Surgical Adjuvant Breast and Bowel Project P-1 Study. *Journal of the National Cancer Institute* 90:1371-88, 1998.

[46] Fisher B., Costantino J. P., Wickerham D. L., Cecchini R. S., Cronin W. M., Robidoux A., et al. Tamoxifen for the prevention of breast cancer: current status of the National Surgical Adjuvant Breast and Bowel Project P-1 study. *Journal of the National Cancer Institute* 97:1652-62, 2005.

[47] Cuzick J., Forbes J. F., Sestak I., Cawthorn S., Hamed H., Holli K., et al. Long-term results of tamoxifen prophylaxis for breast cancer--96-month follow-up of the randomized IBIS-I trial. *Journal of the National Cancer Institute* 99:272-82, 2007.

[48] LaCroix A. Z., Chlebowski R. T., Manson J. A. E., Aragaki A. K., Johnson K. C., Martin L., et al. Health outcomes after stopping conjugated equine estrogens among postmenopausal women with prior hysterectomy. *The Journal of the American Medical Association* 305:1305-514, 2011.

[49] Lewis J. S., Jordan V. C. Case Histories: Raloxifene. In Taylor J and Triggle, D, eds. *Comprehensive Medicinal Chemistry* II, Volume 8 Elsevier Limited, Oxford, U. K. 103-21, 2006.

[50] Jordan V. C. Chemosuppression of breast cancer with tamoxifen: laboratory evidence and future clinical investigations. *Cancer Investigation* 6:589-95, 1988.

[51] Martino S., Cauley J. A., Barrett-Connor E., Powles T. J., Mershon J., Disch D., et al. Continuing outcomes relevant to Evista: breast cancer incidence in postmenopausal osteoporotic women in a randomized trial of raloxifene. *Journal of the National Cancer Institute* 96:1751-61, 2004.

[52] Ettinger B., Black D. M., Mitlak B. H., Knickerbocker R. K., Nickelsen T., Genant H. K., et al. Reduction of vertebral fracture risk in postmenopausal women with osteoporosis treated with raloxifene: results from a 3-year randomized clinical trial. Multiple Outcomes of Raloxifene Evaluation (M. O. R. E.) Investigators. *The Journal of the American Medical Association* 282:637-45, 1999.

[53] Barrett-Connor E., Mosca L., Collins P., Geiger M. J., Grady D., Kornitzer M., et al. Effects of raloxifene on cardiovascular events and breast cancer in postmenopausal women. *The New England Journal of Medicine* 355:125-37, 2006.

[54] Gottardis M. M., Jordan V. C. Development of tamoxifen-stimulated growth of MCF-7 tumors in athymic mice after long-term antiestrogen administration. *Cancer Research* 48:5183-87, 1988.

[55] Wolf D. M., Langan-Fahey S. M., Parker C. J., McCague R., Jordan V. C. Investigation of the mechanism of tamoxifen-stimulated breast tumor growth with nonisomerizable analogues of tamoxifen and metabolites. *Journal of the National Cancer Institute* 85:806-12, 1993.

[56] Yao K., Lee E. S., Bentrem D. J., England G., Schafer J. I. M. G., O'Regan R. M., et al. Antitumor action of physiological estradiol on tamoxifen-stimulated breast tumors grown in athymic mice. *Clinical Cancer Research* 6:2028-36, 2000.

[57] Schafer J. M. G., Lee E. S., O'Regan R. M., Yao K., Jordan V. C. Rapid development of tamoxifen-stimulated mutant p53 breast tumors (T47D) in athymic mice. *Clinical Cancer Research* 6:4373-80, 2000.

[58] Osipo C., Meeke K., Liu H., Cheng D., Lim S., Weichel A., et al. Trastuzumab therapy for tamoxifen-stimulated endometrial cancer. *Cancer Research* 65:8504-13, 2005.

[59] Gottardis M. M., Jiang S. Y., Jeng M. H., Jordan V. C. Inhibition of tamoxifen-stimulated growth of an MCF-7 tumor variant in athymic mice by novel steroidal antiestrogens. *Cancer Research* 49:4090-93, 1989.

[60] Osborne C. K., Coronado-Heinsohn E. B., Hilsenbeck S. G., McCue B. L., Wakeling A. E., McCleland R. A., et al. Comparison of the effects of a pure steroidal antiestrogen with those of tamoxifen in a model of human breast cancer. *Journal of the National Cancer Institute* 87:746-50, 1995.

[61] Lee E. S., Schafer J. M. G., Yao K., England G., O'Regan R. M., De Los Reyes A., et al. Cross-resistance of triphenylethylene-type antiestrogens but not I. C. I. 182,780 in tamoxifen-stimulated breast tumors grown in athymic mice. *Clinical Cancer Research* 6:4893-99, 2000.

[62] Osborne C., Pippen J., Jones S., Parker L., Ellis M., Come S., et al. Double-blind, randomized trial comparing the efficacy and tolerability of fulvestrant versus anastrozole in postmenopausal women with advanced breast cancer progressing on prior endocrine therapy: results of a North American trial. *Journal of Clinical Oncology* 20:3386-95, 2002.

[63] Howell A., Robertson J. F. R., Albano J. Q., Aschermannova A., Mauriac L., Kleeberg U. R., et al. Fulvestrant, formerly I. C. I. 182,780, is as effective as anastrozole in postmenopausal women with advanced breast cancer progressing after prior endocrine treatment. *Journal of Clinical Oncology* 20:3396-403, 2002.

[64] Kent Osborne C., Coronado E. B., Robinson J. P. Human breast cancer in the athymic nude mouse: Cystostatic effects of long-term antiestrogen therapy. *European Journal of Cancer and Clinical Oncology* 23:1189-96, 1987.

[65] Wolf D. M., Jordan V. C. A laboratory model to explain the survival advantage observed in patients taking adjuvant tamoxifen therapy. *Recent results in cancer research Fortschritte der Krebsforschung Progres dans les recherches sur le cancer* 127:23-33, 1993.

[66] Liu H., Lee E. S., Gajdos C., Pearce S. T., Chen B., Osipo C., et al. Apoptotic action of 17β-estradiol in raloxifene-resistant MCF-7 cells in vitro and in vivo. *Journal of the National Cancer Institute* 95:1586-97, 2003.

[67] Balaburski G. M., Dardes R. C., Johnson M., Haddad B., Zhu F., Ross E. A., et al. Raloxifene stimulated experimental breast cancer with the paradoxical actions of estrogen to promote or prevent tumor growth: A Unifying Concept in Antihormone Resistance. *International Journal of Oncology* 37:387-98, 2010.

[68] Lewis J. S., Meeke K., Osipo C., Ross E. A., Kidawi N., Li T., et al. Intrinsic mechanism of estradiol-induced apoptosis in breast cancer cells resistant to estrogen deprivation. *Journal of the National Cancer Institute* 97:1746-59, 2005.

[69] Pink J. J., Jiang S. Y., Fritsch M., Jordan V. C. An estrogen-independent MCF-7 breast cancer cell line which contains a novel 80-kilodalton estrogen receptor-related protein. *Cancer Research* 55:2583-90, 1995.

[70] Jiang S. Y., Wolf D. M., Yingling J. M., Chang C., Jordan V. C. An estrogen receptor positive MCF-7 clone that is resistant to antiestrogens and estradiol. *Molecular and Cellular Endocrinology* 90:77-86, 1992.

[71] Song R. X. D., Mor G., Naftolin F., McPherson R. A., Song J., hang Z., et al. Effect of long-term estrogen deprivation on apoptotic responses of breast cancer cells to 17β-estradiol. *Journal of the National Cancer Institute* 93:1714-23, 2001.

[72] Lewis J., Osipo C., Meeke K., Jordan V. Estrogen-induced apoptosis in a breast cancer model resistant to long-term estrogen withdrawal. The *Journal of steroid biochemistry and molecular biology* 94:131-41, 2005.

[73] Yager J. D., Davidson N. E. Estrogen carcinogenesis in breast cancer. *New England Journal of Medicine* 354:270-82, 2006.

[74] Levenson A. S., Jordan V. C. MCF-7: the first hormone-responsive breast cancer cell line. *Cancer Research* 57:3071-78, 1997.

[75] Jordan V. C. A century of deciphering the control mechanisms of sex steroid action in breast and prostate cancer: the origins of targeted therapy and chemoprevention. *Cancer Research* 69:1243-54, 2009.

[76] Anderson G. L., Chlebowski R. T., Aragaki A. K., Kuller L. H., Manson J. A. E., Gass M., et al. Conjugated equine oestrogen and breast cancer incidence and mortality in postmenopausal women with hysterectomy: extended follow-up of the Women's Health Initiative randomised placebo-controlled trial. *The Lancet Oncology* [epublished ahead of print]:2012.

[77] Jordan V. C. The 38th David A. Karnofsky Lecture: The Paradoxical Actions of Estrogen in Breast Cancer—Survival or Death? *Journal of Clinical Oncology* 26:3073-82, 2008.

[78] Ingle J. N., Ahmann D. L., Green S. J., Edmonson J. H., Bisel H. F., Kvols L. K., et al. Randomized clinical trial of diethylstilbestrol versus tamoxifen in postmenopausal women with advanced breast cancer. *New England Journal of Medicine* 304: 16-21, 1981.

[79] Peethambaram P. P., Ingle J. N., Suman V. J., Hartmann L. C., Loprinzi C. L. Randomized trial of diethylstilbestrol vs. tamoxifen in postmenopausal women with metastatic breast cancer. An updated analysis. *Breast Cancer Research and Treatment* 54:117-22, 1999.

[80] Brünner N., Spang-Thomsen M., Vindeløv L., Nielsen A. Effect of 17 beta-oestradiol on growth curves and flow cytometric D. N. A. distribution of two human breast carcinomas grown in nude mice. *British Journal of Cancer* 47:641-47, 1983.

[81] Brünner N., Bastert G., Poulsen H., Spang-Thomsen M., Engelholm S., Vindeløv L., et al. Characterization of the T61 human breast carcinoma established in nude mice. *European Journal of Cancer and Clinical Oncology* 21:833-43, 1985.

[82] Osipo C., Gajdos C., Liu H., Chen B., Jordan V. C. Paradoxical action of fulvestrant in estradiol-induced regression of tamoxifen-stimulated breast cancer. *Journal of the National Cancer Institute* 95:1597-608, 2003.

[83] Jordan V. C., Liu H., Dardes R. Re: Effect of Long-Term Estrogen Deprivation on Apoptotic Responses of Breast Cancer Cells to 17β-Estradiol and The Two Faces of Janus: Sex Steroids as Mediators of Both Cell Proliferation and Cell Death. *Journal of the National Cancer Institute* 94:1173-75, 2002.

[84] Chisamore M. J., Ahmed Y., Bentrem D. J., Jordan V. C., Tonetti D. A. Novel Antitumor Effect of Estradiol in Athymic Mice Injected with a T47D Breast Cancer Cell Line Overexpressing Protein Kinase Cα. *Clinical Cancer Research* 7:3156-65, 2001.

[85] Osipo C., Meeke K., Cheng D., Weichel A., Bertucci A., Hong L., et al. Role for HER2/neu and HER3 in fulvestrant-resistant breast cancer. *International Journal of Oncology* 30:509-20, 2007.

[86] Song R. X. D., Zhang Z., Mor G., Santen R. Down-regulation of Bcl-2 enhances estrogen apoptotic action in long-term estradiol-depleted ER+ breast cancer cells. *Apoptosis* 10:667-78, 2005.

[87] Ariazi E. A., Cunliffe H. E., Lewis-Wambi J. S., Slifker M. J., Willis A. L., Ramos P., et al. Estrogen induces apoptosis in estrogen deprivation-resistant breast cancer through stress responses as identified by global gene expression across time. *Proceedings of the National Academy of Sciences* 108:18879-86, 2011.

[88] Maximov P., Sengupta S., Lewis-Wambi J. S., Kim H. R., Curpan R. F., Jordan V. C. The Conformation of the Estrogen Receptor Directs Estrogen-Induced Apoptosis in Breast Cancer: A Hypothesis. *Hormone molecular biology and clinical investigation* 5:27-34, 2011.

[89] Obiorah I., Sengupta S., Curpan R., Jordan V. Alteration of the shape of the ligand estrogen receptor complex controls estrogen induced apoptosis in breast cancer [abstract number 3924]. Proceedings of the 103rd Annual Meeting of the American Association for Cancer Research; Chicago, Illinois, Mar. 31-Apr. 4 2012.

[90] Fan P., Griffith O., Anur P., Kim H., Gray J., Jordan V. Critical Mediation of E2-induced Apoptosis through c-Src in Long-term Estrogen Deprived Breast Cancer Cells. Minisymposium of steroid hormone receptors in breast and prostate cancer [abstract number 2921]. A. A. C. R. annual meeting; Chicago, Illinois, Mar. 31-Apr. 4 2012.

[91] Ali S., Coombes R. C. Endocrine-responsive breast cancer and strategies for combating resistance. *Nature Reviews Cancer* 2:101-12, 2002.

[92] Lønning P. E., Taylor P. D., Anker G., Iddon J., Wie L., Jørgensen L. M., et al. High-dose estrogen treatment in postmenopausal breast cancer patients heavily exposed to endocrine therapy. *Breast Cancer Research and Treatment* 67:111-16, 2001.

[93] Lønning P. E. Additive endocrine therapy for advanced breast cancer-back to the future. *Acta Oncologica* 48:1092-101, 2009.

[94] Ellis M. J., Gao F., Dehdashti F., Jeffe D. B., Marcom P. K., Carey L. A., et al. Lower-Dose vs High-Dose Oral Estradiol Therapy of Hormone Receptor–Positive, Aromatase Inhibitor–Resistant Advanced Breast Cancer. *The Journal of the American Medical Association* 302:774-80, 2009.

[95] Stefanick M. L., Anderson G. L., Margolis K. L., Hendrix S. L., Rodabough R. J., Paskett E. D., et al. Effects of conjugated equine estrogens on breast cancer and mammography screening in postmenopausal women with hysterectomy. *The Journal of the American Medical Association* 295:1647-57, 2006.

[96] Prentice R. L., Chlebowski R. T., Stefanick M. L., Manson J. A. E., Langer R. D., Pettinger M., et al. Conjugated equine estrogens and breast cancer risk in the Women's Health Initiative clinical trial and observational study. *American Journal of Epidemiology* 167:1407-15, 2008.

[97] Willis D. B., Calle E. E., Miracle-McMahill H. L., Heath C. W. Estrogen replacement therapy and risk of fatal breast cancer in a prospective cohort of postmenopausal women in the United States. *Cancer Causes and Control* 7:449-57, 1996.

[98] Chlebowski R. T., Anderson G. L., Gass M., Lane D. S., Aragaki A. K., Kuller L. H., et al. Estrogen plus progestin and breast cancer incidence and mortality in postmenopausal women. *The Journal of the American Medical Association* 304:1684-92, 2010.

[99] Chlebowski R. T., Anderson G. L., Manson J. E., Schwartz A. G., Wakelee H., Gass M., et al. Lung Cancer Among Postmenopausal Women Treated With Estrogen Alone in the Women's Health Initiative Randomized Trial. *Journal of the National Cancer Institute* 102:1413-21, 2010.

[100] Jordan V. C., Ford L. G. Paradoxical Clinical Effect of Estrogen on Breast Cancer Risk: A "New" Biology of Estrogen-induced Apoptosis. *Cancer Prevention Research* 4:633-37, 2011.

[101] Welshons W. V., Jordan V. C. Adaptation of estrogen-dependent MCF-7 cells to low estrogen (phenol red-free) culture. European *Journal of Cancer and Clinical Oncology* 23:1935-39, 1987.

[102] Vogel V. G., Costantino J. P., Wickerham D. L., Cronin W. M., Cecchini R. S., Atkins J. N., et al. Update of the national surgical adjuvant breast and bowel project study of tamoxifen and raloxifene (STAR) P-2 trial: preventing breast cancer. *Cancer Prevention Research* 3:696-706, 2010.

Index

C

D

E

F

G

H

P

Q

R

S

W

X

Y